Springer Tracts in Advanced Robotics

Volume 69

Editors: Bruno Siciliano · Oussama Khatib · Frans Groen

Eduardo Rocon and José L. Pons

Exoskeletons in Rehabilitation Robotics

Tremor Suppression

Springer

Professor Bruno Siciliano, Dipartimento di Informatica e Sistemistica, Università di Napoli Federico II, Via Claudio 21, 80125 Napoli, Italy, E-mail: siciliano@unina.it

Professor Oussama Khatib, Artificial Intelligence Laboratory, Department of Computer Science, Stanford University, Stanford, CA 94305-9010, USA, E-mail: khatib@cs.stanford.edu

Professor Frans Groen, Department of Computer Science, Universiteit van Amsterdam, Kruislaan 403, 1098 SJ Amsterdam, The Netherlands, E-mail: groen@science.uva.nl

Authors

Dr. Eduardo Rocon
Biongineering group, IAI-CSIC
Ctra. Campo Real, km 0.200
La Poveda - Arganda del Rey
28500 Madrid, Spain
E-mail: erocon@iai.csic.es

Dr. José L. Pons
Biongineering group, IAI-CSIC
Ctra. Campo Real, km 0.200
La Poveda - Arganda del Rey
28500 Madrid, Spain
E-mail: jlpons@iai.csic.es

ISBN 978-3-642-17658-6 e-ISBN 978-3-642-17659-3

DOI 10.1007/978-3-642-17659-3

Springer Tracts in Advanced Robotics ISSN 1610-7438

Typeset & Cover Design: Scientific Publishing Services Pvt. Ltd., Chennai, India.

Printed on acid-free paper

5 4 3 2 1 0

springer.com

STAR (Springer Tracts in Advanced Robotics) has been promoted under the auspices of EURON (European Robotics Research Network)

To our families

Foreword

Robotics is undergoing a major transformation in scope and dimension. From a largely dominant industrial focus, robotics is rapidly expanding into human environments and vigorously engaged in its new challenges. Interacting with, assisting, serving, and exploring with humans, the emerging robots will increasingly touch people and their lives.

Beyond its impact on physical robots, the body of knowledge robotics has produced is revealing a much wider range of applications reaching across diverse research areas and scientific disciplines, such as: biomechanics, haptics, neurosciences, virtual simulation, animation, surgery, and sensor networks among others. In return, the challenges of the new emerging areas are proving an abundant source of stimulation and insights for the field of robotics. It is indeed at the intersection of disciplines that the most striking advances happen.

The Springer Tracts in Advanced Robotics (STAR) is devoted to bringing to the research community the latest advances in the robotics field on the basis of their significance and quality. Through a wide and timely dissemination of critical research developments in robotics, our objective with this series is to promote more exchanges and collaborations among the researchers in the community and contribute to further advancements in this rapidly growing field.

The monograph written by Eduardo Rocon and José Pons is a contribution in the area of rehabilitation robotics, which has been receiving a growing deal of attention by the research community in the latest few years. The contents are focused on the management and suppression of pathological tremor in upper limb exoskeletons. Solutions deal with both cognitive and physical human-robot interaction issues of such wearable devices. Results are validated in a rich set of experiments, revealing a promising outlook toward the application to a wide range of so-called soft robots.

Remarkably, the monograph is based on the first author's doctoral thesis, which received the prize of the Seventh Edition of the EURON Georges Giralt PhD Award devoted to the best PhD thesis in Robotics in Europe. A very fine addition to STAR!

Naples, Italy
September 2010

Bruno Siciliano
STAR Editor

Preface

The scientific community is becoming more and more interested in rehabilitation robotics. From a robotics perspective, exoskeletons are mechatronic systems worn by a person in such a way that the physical interface leads to a direct transfer of mechanical power and exchange of information. A wearable robot is designed to match the shape and function of the human body. Segments and joints correspond to some extent to those of the human body while the system is externally coupled to the person. Initially, the primary applications of these robotic mechanisms were teleoperation and power amplification. Later, exoskeletons have been considered as rehabilitation and assistive devices for disabled or elderly people. One important and specific feature of wearable robotics is the intrinsic interaction between human and robot. This interaction is twofolded: first, cognitive, because the human controls the robot while it provides feedback to the human; secondly, a biomechanical interaction leading to the application of controlled forces between both actors.

The fact that a human being is an integral part of the design is one of the most exciting and challenging aspects in the design of biomechatronics wearable robots. It imposes several restrictions and requirements in the design of this sort of devices.

Tremor is characterized by involuntary oscillations of a part of the body. The most accepted definition is as follows: "an involuntary, approximately rhythmic, and roughly sinusoidal movement". Tremor is a disabling consequence of a number of neurological disorders. Tremor, the most common of all involuntary movements, can affect various body parts such as the hands, head, facial structures, tongue, trunk, and legs. Most tremors, however, occur in the hands. Tremor is a disorder that is not life-threatening, but it can be responsible for functional disability and social inconvenience. More than 65% of the population with upper limb tremor have serious difficulties performing daily living activities. In many cases, tremor intensities are very large, causing total disability to the affected person. The overall management of tremor is directed towards keeping the patient functioning independently as long as possible while minimizing disability.

It has been established in the literature that most of the different types of tremor respond to biomechanical loading. In particular, it has been clinically tested that the increase of damping and/or inertia in the upper limb leads to a reduction of the tremorous motion. This phenomenon gives rise to the possibility of an orthotic management of tremor. An orthosis is a wearable device that acts in parallel to the affected limb. In the case of tremor management, the orthosis must apply a damping or inertial load to a selected set of limb articulations. As a wearable device, it must exhibit a number of aesthetic and functional characteristics. Aesthetics is more directly related to size, weight and appearance of the exoskeleton. Functionality is related to generating required torque and velocity while maintaining the robustness of operation.

This book will give a general overview of the robotic exoskeletons field and will introduce the reader to this new robotic field with an extensive review of its main applications and the technologies suitable for its development. In addition, it provides detailed studies of the main topics in the wearable robotics field. The book will use the development of an upper limb exoskeleton for tremor suppression in order to illustrate the influence of a specific application in the designs decisions. It will present the development and validation of an upper limb exoskeleton with three main objectives: monitoring and diagnosis, and validation of non-grounded tremor reduction strategies.

At the end, the book focuses on describing the upcoming research in the rehabilitation field which leads to the concept of Soft-Robots (SRs). They are also wearable, but SRs use functional human structures instead of artificial counterparts, e.g. artificial actuators are substituted by Functional Electrical Stimulation (FES) of human muscles. The borderline between human and robot becomes fuzzy and this immediatilly leads to hybrid Human-Robot systems.

Madrid, September 2010

Eduardo Rocon
José L. Pons

Acknowledgements

The work presented in this paper has been carried out with the financial support from the Commission of the European Union, within Framework 5, specific RTD programme “Quality of Life and Management of Living Resources”, Key Action 6.4 “Aging and Disabilities”, under Contract QKL6-CT-2002-00536, “DRIFTS - Dynamically Responsive Intervention for Tremor Suppression.” The future work defined in the book is ongoing at the Bioengineering Group, CSIC. These activities are part of a large-scale project called HYPER which is funded by CONSOLIDER- INGENIO Research supported by CONSOLIDER-INGENIO 2010 Programme of the Spanish Ministry of Science and Innovation, (grant CSD2009-00067). However, in the particular scenario of tremor suppression ongoing research activities are being carried out in the framework of the European project TREMOR with the financial support from the Commission of the European Union, within Framework 7, specific IST programme “Accessible and Inclusive ICT”, Target outcome 7.2 “Advanced self-adaptive ICT-enabled assistive systems based on non-invasive Brain to Computer Interaction (BCI) ”, under Grant Agreement number ICT-2007-224051, “TREMOR. An ambulatory BCI-driven tremor suppression system based on functional electrical stimulation.”

We wish to express our gratitude to the consorsotium of DRIFTS and TREMOR projects, in particular to Lawrence Normie, Juan Manuel-Belda Lois and Andrés Felipe Ruiz Olaya.

The writing of this book would have not been possible without help and contribution of all our colleagues at CSIC, in particular to the Bioengineering Group headed by Prof. Ramón Ceres.

Finally, we would like to thank Prof. Bruno Siciliano for encouraging and giving us the opportunity to write this book.

Contents

1 Introduction: Exoskeletons in Rehabilitation Robotics ... 1

1.1 Introduction to Rehabilitation Robotics: Tremor Management ... 1

1.2 Historical Note on Rehabilitation Robotics ... 5

1.3 The Role of Robotic Exoskeletons in Rehabilitation ... 7

1.4 Salient Issues in Exoskeletal Rehabilitation Robotics ... 10

1.4.1 Bioinspiration ... 12

1.4.2 Mechanisms and Dynamic Models ... 13

1.4.3 Physical HRI in the Context of Exoskeletal Robots ... 13

1.4.4 Cognitive HMI in the Context of Exoskeletal Robots ... 14

1.4.5 Sensors, Actuators and Supporting Technologies ... 16

1.5 Scope of the Book ... 16

2 Pathological Tremor Management ... 21

2.1 Introduction ... 21

2.2 Tremor Manifestations ... 22

2.3 Tremor Patterns ... 24

2.3.1 Essential Tremor ... 26

2.3.2 Parkinsonian tremor ... 27

2.3.3 Cerebellar tremor ... 28

2.4 Tremor Characterization at Joint Level ... 29

2.4.1 Measuring Tremor: The Experimental Protocol ... 31

2.4.2 Studying Tremor: The Hilbert Spectrum ... 35

2.4.3 Tremor Study Based on Empirical Mode Decomposition ... 45

2.4.4 Study of Tremor Characteristics Based on a Biomechanical Model of the Upper Limb ... 46

2.5 Conclusions ... 50

3 Upper Limb Exoskeleton for Tremor Suppression: Cognitive HR Interaction . . . 53
3.1 Tremor Isolation . . . 54
3.2 Estimation of Voluntary Movement . . . 55
3.2.1 Two Points Extrapolator . . . 57
3.2.2 g-h Filters . . . 57
3.2.3 The Kalman Filter . . . 61
3.2.4 Figure of Merit . . . 63
3.3 Real-Time Estimation of Voluntary and Tremorous Movement . . . 64
3.4 Conclusions . . . 65

4 Upper Limb Exoskeleton for Tremor Suppression: Physical HR Interaction . . . 67
4.1 Biomechanics of the Upper Limb . . . 68
4.1.1 Tolerance to Pressure . . . 68
4.1.2 Mechanical Characterization of Soft Tissues at the Upper-Limb . . . 69
4.2 Wearable Orthosis for Tremor Assessment and Suppression, WOTAS . . . 71
4.2.1 Mechanical Design . . . 71
4.2.2 Sensors . . . 74
4.2.3 Actuators . . . 75
4.3 Control Architecture . . . 77
4.4 Control Strategies for Tremor Suppression . . . 78
4.4.1 Tremor Reduction through Impedance Control . . . 80
4.4.2 Exploitation of the Repetitive Characteristics of Tremor Movement . . . 90
4.5 Conclusions . . . 97

5 Upper Limb Exoskeleton for Tremor Suppression: Validation . . . 99
5.1 Experimental Protocol . . . 99
5.1.1 Users . . . 99
5.1.2 Materials and Methods . . . 100
5.1.3 Tasks . . . 101
5.1.4 Data Analysis . . . 102
5.2 Results and Discussion . . . 102
5.3 Discussion . . . 108
5.4 Conclusions . . . 110

6 Summary, Conclusions and Upcoming Research 113
6.1 Summary 113
6.2 Conclusions 116
6.3 Upcoming Research 117
6.3.1 Development of Algorithms to Identify Intention to Move 125
6.3.2 Development of Algorithms to Identify Tremor Onset 125
6.3.3 Development of Algorithms for Tracking and Extraction of Tremor Characteristics 127
References 131

Chapter 1
Introduction: Exoskeletons in Rehabilitation Robotics

1.1 Introduction to Rehabilitation Robotics: Tremor Management

Rehabilitation Robotics has been defined as the combination of industrial robotics and medical rehabilitation, thus encompassing many areas, including mechanical and electrical engineering, biomedical engineering, artificial intelligence and sensor and actuator technology. Medical rehabilitation often refers to the process by which human function, be it physical or cognitive, is restored at least partially to their "normal" condition.

Strictly speaking, Rehabilitation Robotics would not encompass systems that aim at replacing the mechanical function of weak or missing human limbs. However, in an integrative view, here we also consider functional restoration as an important area within Rehabilitation Robotics. As a consequence, all four wearable robots depicted in figure 1.1 are considered here true rehabilitation robots.

Therefore the objective of Rehabilitation Robotics can be stated as the application of robotics to assist the user to function with a maximum of autonomy. The ideal situation arrives when, by means of the assistive rehabilitation robot, [74]:

- The user is autonomous in the execution of a given task;
- The user is able to function in daily life with less human assistance;
- The user either has his physical or cognitive functions restored or is able to function for a number of hours with the assistance of the robotic companion and without human assistance.

This ideal scenario usually is to be met by a combination of a rehabilitation robot and an environment modification. This goes in line with [74], where assistive devices are not limited to the robotic system but consist of a system of compatible devices which communicate among them. This approach integrates users into a comprehensive system in which they are in control of the rehabilitation robot, any other mobility system and they can exert control on the environment whenever it is not fully provided by the robotic device. In more recent approaches, [9], the robotic assistant mediates between the user and all these environmental controls. A clear

E. Rocon and J.L. Pons: Exoskeletons in Rehabilitation Robotics, STAR 69, pp. 1–20.
springerlink.com

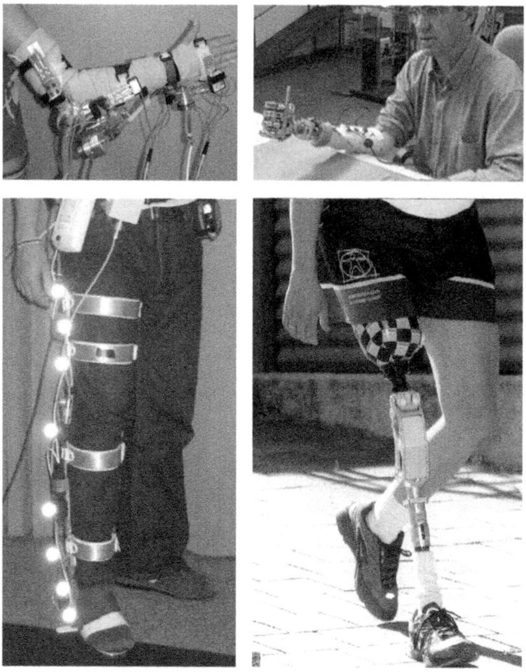

Fig. 1.1 Wearable robots: (top left) an upper limb orthotic exoskeleton; (top right) an upper limb prosthetic robot; (bottom left) a lower limb orthotic exoskeleton; (bottom right) a lower limb prosthetic robot.

example of this approach is shown along this book. A robotic system is developed for the purpose of suppressing pathological tremor. Some of the technologies specifically developed and integrated in the robotic exoskeletal structure are then used to modify the environment, e.g. algorithms to detect tremor are integrated in computer filters so that users can interact with them via input peripherals (e.g. mouse or joystick).

There is a clear global trend towards ageing, [72]. According to the World Health Organization (WHO), elderly population (65+) will increase by roughly 90% in the coming years. This will take the contingent of senior citizens in US by 2050 to 80 million, similar figures are expected in Europe. This global trend represents an opportunity to develop and deploy assistive technologies such as rehabilitation robots.

Rehabilitation robots can be conceived as (1) fixed-base or end-effector systems and as (2) exoskeleton systems. According to Krebs, [72], the decision on what particular approach is to be used is based on kinematics criteria and depends mostly on the application and, in particular, on the motion ranges the system allows to the human limbs. It is claimed that for limb segment movements requiring less that 45 degrees end-effector system appear more appropriate. On the other hand, exoskeletal structures are more appropriate for larger limb joint excursions. This decision is also to be taken based on ambulatory and portability issues. Whenever a portable solution is expected, exoskeletal structures are likely more convenient.

The choice between end-effector and exoskeleton structures has major implications on the design of the rehabilitation system. Both end-effector and exoskeletal systems are in close physical interaction with the human user, however exoskeletons exhibit continuous and multipoint physical interaction which is mediated through users' soft tissues and they typically map onto several human anatomical joints which leads to potential kinematic incompatibility and undesired interactions. For an exhaustive analysis of exoskeletons the reader is referred to [95].

Along this book we will analyze the application of rehabilitation robots, in particular exoskeletal structures, for the active management of tremor suppression via portable robotics. Tremor is a symptom of various neurological conditions. There is no known cure for several tremor diseases. The overall management is direct toward keeping the patient functioning independently as long as possible while minimizing disability. In view of what is currently known, the treatment options available for tremor are medication, neurosurgical intervention, rehabilitation programs (psychotherapy), brain stimulation, and assistance to the limb with compensatory technology.

The standard and most effective treatment of tremor is medication. One of the main issues here is that drugs are typically prescribed on a trial-and-error basis in order of decreasing expected effectiveness because the clinical phenomenological tremor classifications are not perfectly predictive of their success. If success in reducing tremor is attained, it must be weighed against side effects and the potential for addiction, [2].

Drug therapies have not been very successful in tremor treatment, giving rise to the need of alternative approaches to the problem of tremor suppression. For those cases in which there is no effective drug treatment, physical interventions such as teaching the patient to brace the affected limb during the tremor are sometimes useful. The goals of rehabilitation program include preservation of present function, improve range of motion, posture, strength, and endurance; prevention of disabling complications (e.g., respiratory, bowel, bladder, visual); family training; and maintenance of the patient's independence as long as possible.

More recently, there has been research interest in the use of deep brain stimulation of the globus pallidus or subthalamic nucleus as a treatment of people that suffer of tremor diseases, specially of some Parkinsonian symptoms, such as rigidity, bradykinesia, or akinesia. Caparros, [21], in his work discovered that high-frequency electrical stimulation of ventralis intermedius suppresses Parkinson tremor, and Friston, [41], stated that the suppression of tremor is associated to reduced blood flow in the cerebellum. A commercial example of this approach is the Medtronic Activa Tremor Control System. The Activa Tremor Control System (Medtronic Corp., Minnesota) has been approved by the FDA (Food and Drug Administration - U.S. Department of Healthy and Human Services) for "unilateral thalamic stimulation for the suppression of tremor in the upper extremity in patients who are diagnosed with essential tremor or Parkinsonian tremor not adequately controlled by medications and where the tremor constitutes a significant functional disability".

The main drawbacks of these treatments are:

1. tremor is not managed effectively and sufficiently in about 25% of patients, [15],
2. the drugs used often induce side effects or may be contra-indicated, [135],
3. surgery is associated with a risk of haemorrhage and psychiatric manifestations, [17]. In particular, a high rate of suicide (4.3%) has been observed recently in patients treated with deep brain stimulation, [20].

As a consequence, further research and new therapeutic options are required to manage tremor more effectively. It has been established in the literature that most of the different types of tremor respond to mechanical loading of the affected limb, [1, 71, 89]. In particular, it has been clinically tested that the increase of damping and/or inertia in the upper limb leads to a reduction of the tremorous motion, [1]. This phenomenon, i.e. the change in impedance characteristics of the upper limb, has a direct effect on the tremor characteristics and gives rise to the possibility of an orthotic management of tremor.

Biomechanical loading for tremor reduction can be approached either by exoskeletal robotics or by non-ambulatory, table or wheelchair mounted, end-effector devices. The former approach is characterized by selective tremor suppression through internal forces (i.e. forces applied between consecutive segments in the upper limb kinematic chain) at particular joints, while the latter relies on global application of external forces that leads to the overall tremor reduction.

While wearable tremor suppression exoskeletons are already a matter of research, non-ambulatory systems have lead to commercial products, see, for instance, the so-called Neater Eater, [89]. In addition, the MIT damped joystick, [52], the controlled Energy-Dissipation Orthosis, CEDO, [116], or the Modulated Energy Dissipation Arm, MED, (cited in [71]), are implementations of non-ambulatory, wheelchair-mounted tremor suppression prototypes.

As far as wearable tremor suppression concepts are concerned, just the well-know wearable tremor-suppression orthosis, [71], has been reported in literature. This is a semi-active damping loading device, which acts mechanically in parallel to the wrist in flexion-extension. It completely constrains both wrist abduction-adduction and pronation-supination.

In the framework of the DRIFTS (dynamically responsive intervention for tremor suppression) project, [81], the WOTAS exoskeleton was presented as an alternative treatment for tremor. The exoskeleton was developed with three main objectives: monitoring, diagnosis, and validation of ungrounded tremor reduction strategies. An exoskeleton is a wearable device that acts in parallel to the affected limb. In the case of tremor management, it must apply a damping or inertial load to a selected set of limb articulations. As a wearable device, it must exhibit a number of aesthetic and functional characteristics. Aesthetics is more directly related to size, weight and appearance of the exoskeleton. Functionality is related to generating required torque and velocity while maintaining the robustness of operation. This book will present the development and validation of such a platform and at the end the conclusions and future trends of this study are given.

1.2 Historical Note on Rehabilitation Robotics

Rehabilitation Robotics is not a new discipline. Rehabilitation Robotics has evolved along the last 5 decades starting from pioneering work at Case Institute of Technology in the early 1960's, ever since work on rehabilitation robots has been continued in parallel in U.S., [50], and Europe, [26]. In this section, we will briefly review main milestones in research on rehabilitation robots.

Rehabilitation Robotics first started in North America. First instances of rehabilitation robots in U.S. comprise the floor mounted, four degrees-of-freedom, externally powered exoskeleton developed at Case Institute of Technology in early 1960's, the so-called Rancho Golden arm which is a six degrees-of-freedom powered orthosis developed in 1969 at Rancho Los Amigos Hospital, the Johns Hopkins arm consisting in a four degrees-of-freedom arm plus hand and the use of RTX robot prototype at Boeing to deal with book and paper handling.

Amongst all these pioneering research activities it is worth highlighting the joint U.S. Department of Veterans Affairs and Stanford University (VA/SU) Robotics program that extended over a period of more than 15 years on the topic of rehabilitation robots. The program started with the Robotics Aid Project (RAP) between 1978 and 1985. The goal of this project was to use industrial robots in combination with prototype user interface devices to derive a system usable by persons affected by quadriplegia, [133]. In this first project, the robot could be voice-controlled in various different coordinate systems. In this way the user was able to command preexisting robot programs. A second project in the framework of the VA/SU Robotics program was the Clinical Robotics Laboratory (CRL) project which was active between 1985 and 1989. The Clinical Robotics Laboratory was established in the VA Spinal Cord Injury Center (SCIC) for development and evaluation of a new generation of robots assisting people in Activities of Daily Living (ADLs). Again, industrial robots (a new generation, the PUMA-260 this time) was adapted to the task.

While in the previous two projects the concept of the desktop assistant was explored, the next project in the series, the so-called Mobile Vocational Assistant Robot (MoVAR), 1983-1988 used a new three-wheeled omnidirectional base with a PUMA-250 arm mounted on it. This time the system was designed desk-high and had the ability of going through interior doorways. All the components, electronics and power, were mounted in the mobile base. A telemetry system between the console and the robot allowed the transmission of position and status information. The system interfaces with the patients using either voice control, a keyboard or head-motion inputs. A desktop version of the MoVAR assistant was the object of the next research project, the Desktop Vocational Assistant Robot (DeVAR), 1989-1994. The concept of the vocationally oriented workstations was retaken with the aim of addressing target areas for which reimbursement of capital equipment would be possible, [133]. The idea is that assistive technology in the vocational domain would be an incentive for people with severe physical disabilities return to the workforce.

Very important conclusions were derived from the VA/SU Rehabilitation Robotics program:

- The concept of considering the person with a disability "the" user of the rehabilitation robot must be reconsidered. When the whole value chain of the rehabilitation robot is considered, then it becomes apparent that the therapists, will be mainly concerned with the interface layer of the rehabilitation robot (as they will have to use hardware and software tools for a proper adjustment, set-up and customization), physicians will use robot-generated reports to assess how the therapy is evolving, and finally hospital administrations, Health authorities and Insurance companies will be mainly interested in costs and patient outcomes. This leads to the necessity of considering all these multiple users along the conceptualization, design, prototyping and evaluation of rehabilitation robots.
- The importance of robot-based Clinical Evaluation Tools. During the VA/SU program it was apparent that the involvement of clinical personnel, hand-in-hand with engineers, was crucial. The program developed several robot-based evaluation tools (e.g. history list feature) to support the evaluation of systems and users' evolution. This topic together with the previous one leads to the need that users (patients) and clinicians are tightly involved in the design process of rehabilitation robots.
- The importance of embedding the design process in an iterative design-evaluation cycle so that technology and methodological/evaluation tools are developed in concert.

In parallel to the work at VA/SU, in Canada, the Robotics Assistive Appliance (RAA) was developed at Neil Squire Foundation. The research activities at Neil Squire Foundation resulted in a six degrees-of-freedom robot that was interfaced to the users via a variety of modalities, including sip-and-puff, Morse codes and voice control.

The French project Spartacus can be regarded as one of the first activities on rehabilitation robotics in Europe. Spartacus involved a feasibility study on the use of telemanipulators by people with spinal cord injuries. The project focused on control ergonomics of a workstation configuration based, first, on a MA-23 nuclear telemanipulator and, second, on a custom designed telethesis (MAT-1). In parallel to this work, the Heidelberg Manipulator was sponsored by the German Federal Ministry of Research and Technology. Again, the Heidelberg Manipulator was a workstation-based approach developed from the specifications derived from the statements of 75 tetraplegic individuals, [26].

Both projects jointly with other research activities in North America were brought together in 1978 in an international seminal conference where all research groups active on the topic were present. From this starting point, Rehabilitation Robotics begun to be a permanent topic in more general conferences, first in conferences of the Rehabilitation Engineering and Assistive Technology Society of North America (RESNA), and then Robotics conferences of IEEE. In this regard, the discipline has evolved into mature work groups like the IEEE Robotics and Automation's Technical Committee on Rehabilitation & Assistive Robotics and thematic conferences have been organized along the last decade, e.g. IEEE International Conference on Rehabilitation Robots (ICORR).

1.3 The Role of Robotic Exoskeletons in Rehabilitation

The exoskeleton is a species of wearable robot with very interesting applications in the Rehabilitation arena, [95]. The distinctive, specific and singular aspect of exoskeletons is that the exoskeleton's kinematic chain maps onto the human limb anatomy. There is a one-to-one correspondence between human anatomical joints and the robot's joints or sets of joints. This kinematic compliance is a key aspect in achieving ergonomic human–robot interfaces, as is further illustrated along this book.

In exoskeletons, there is an effective transfer of power between the human and the robot. Humans and exoskeletons are in close physical interaction. This is the reverse of master-slave configurations, where there is no physical contact between the slave and the human operator, which are remote from one another. However, in some instances of teleoperation, an upper-limb exoskeleton can be used as the interface between the human and the remote robot. According to this concept, the exoskeleton can be used as an input device (by establishing a pose correspondence between the human and the slave or remote manipulator), as a force feedback device (by providing haptic interaction between the slave robot and its environment), or both.

Of the different robots, exoskeletons are the ones in which the cognitive (information) and physical (power) interactions with the human operator are most intense. In line with the historical note above introduced, scientific and technological work on exoskeletons began in the early 1960s. The US Department of Defense became interested in developing the concept of a powered "suit of armor". At the same time, at Cornel Aeronautical Laboratories work started to develop the concept of man–amplifiers — manipulators to enhance the strength of a human operator. The existing technological limitations on development of the concept were established in 1962; these related to servos, sensors and mechanical structure and design. Later on, in 1964, the hydraulic actuator technology was identified as an additional limiting factor.

General Electric Co. further developed the concept of human–amplifiers through the *Hardiman project* from 1966 to 1971. The Hardiman concept was more of a robotic master/slave configuration in which two overlapping exoskeletons were implemented. The inner one was set to follow human motion while the outer one implemented a hydraulically powered version of the motion performed by the inner exoskeleton. The concept of extenders versus master/slave robots as systems exhibiting genuine information and power transmission between the two actors was coined in 1990, [69].

Rehabilitation and functional compensation exoskeletons are another classic field of application for wearable robotics. Passive orthotic or prosthetic devices do not fall within the scope of this book, but they may be regarded as the forebears of current rehabilitation exoskeletons. More than a century ago, Prof. H. Wangenstein proposed the concept of a mobility assistant for scientists bereft of the use of their legs:

> "This amazing feat shall revolutionize the way in which paraplegic Scientists continue their honorable work in the advancement of Science! Even in this modern day and age, some injuries cannot be healed. Even with all the Science at our command, some of our learned brethren today are without the use of their legs. This Device will change all that. From an ordinary-appearing wheelchair, the Pneumatic Bodyframe will transform into a light exoskeleton which will allow the Scientist to walk about normally. Even running and jumping are not beyond its capabilities, all controlled by the power of the user's mind. The user simply seats himself in the chair, fits the restraining belts around his chest, waist, thighs and calves, fastens the Neuro-Impulse Recognition Electrodes (N.I.R.E.) to his temples, and is ready to go!"

The concept introduced by Prof. Wangenstein in 1883 contains the main features of current state-of-the-art wearable robotic exoskeletons: a pneumatically actuated body frame (in the form of a light exoskeleton), mapping onto the human lower limb, in which a cHRI is established by means of brain activity electrodes (known as N.I.R.E.).

Among the spinoff applications of robotic extenders are robotic upper limb orthoses, [100]. Although studies on active controlled orthoses date back to the mid 1950s, [11], the first active implementations of powered orthoses were the work of [102]. This functional upper-limb orthosis was conceived for people with limited strength in their arms.

The interaction between the exoskeleton and the human limb can be achieved through *internal force* or *external force* systems. Which of these force interaction concepts is chosen depends chiefly on the application. On the one hand, empowering exoskeletons must be based on the concept of external force systems; empowering exoskeletons are used to multiply the force that a human wearer can withstand, and therefore the force that the environment exerts on the exoskeleton must be grounded: that is, in external force systems the exoskeleton's mechanical structure acts as a load-carrying device and only a small part of the force is exerted on the wearer. The power is transmitted to an external base, be it fixed or portable with the operator. The only power transmission is between the human limbs and the robot as a means of implementing control inputs and/or force feedback. This concept is illustrated in figure 1.3 (right).

On the other hand, orthotic exoskeletons, i.e. exoskeletons for functional compensation of human limbs, work on the internal force principle. In this instance of a wearable robot, the force and power is transmitted by means of the exoskeleton between segments of the human limb. Orthotic exoskeletons are applicable whenever there is weakness or loss of human limb function. In such a scenario, the exoskeleton complements or replaces the function of the human musculoskeletal system. In internal force exoskeletons, the force is non-grounded; force is applied only between the exoskeleton and the limb. The concept of internal force exoskeletons is illustrated in figure 1.3 (left).

Superimposing a robot on a human limb, as in the case of exoskeletons, is a difficult problem. Ideally, the human must feel no restriction to his natural motion

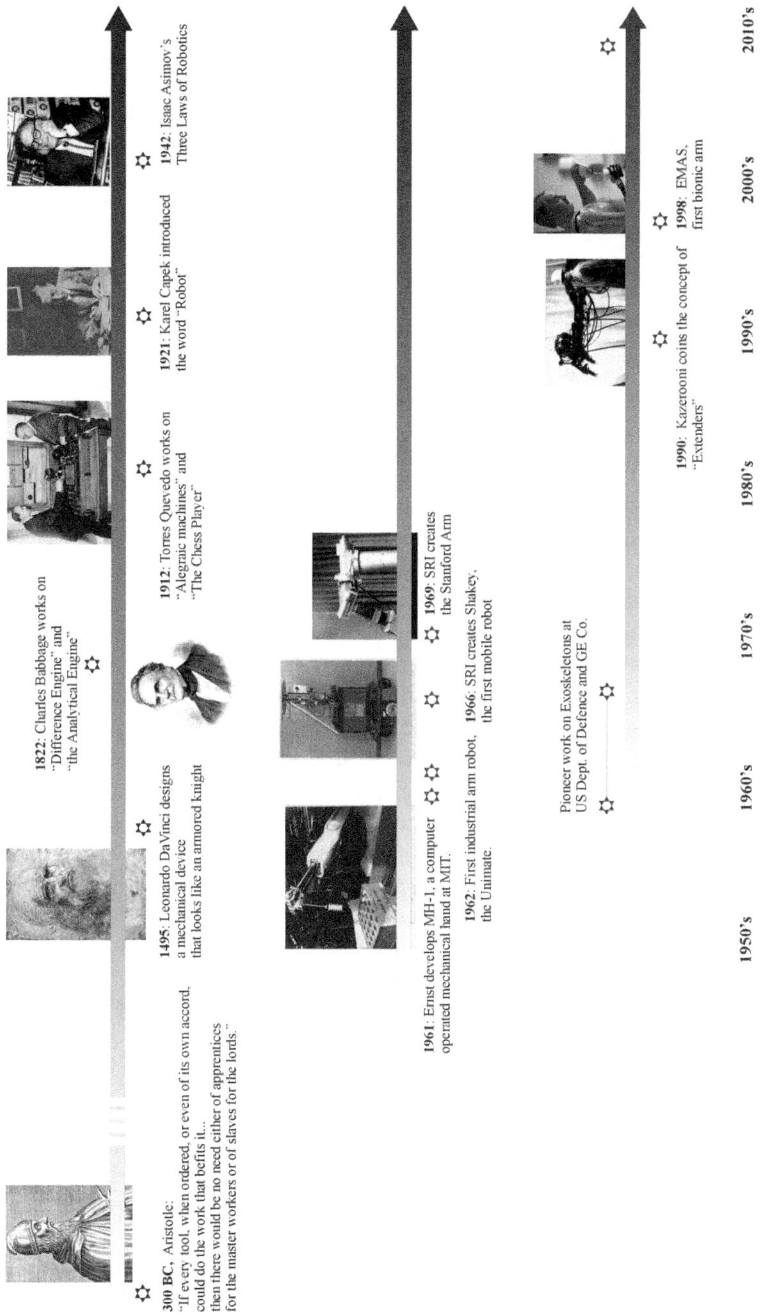

Fig. 1.2 Chronological evolution of Robotics and Wearable Robotics.

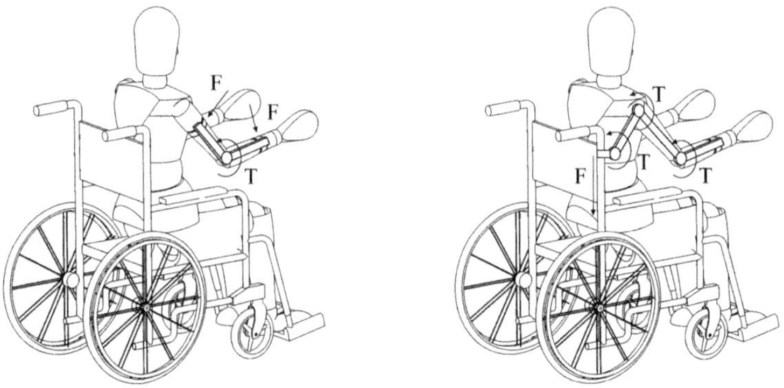

Fig. 1.3 Schematic representation of internal force (left) and external force (right) exoskeletal systems.

patterns. Therefore, kinematics plays a key role in wearable exoskeletons: if robots and humans are not kinematically compliant, a source of non-ergonomic interaction forces appears. This is comprehensively addressed along this book.

Kinematic compatibility is of paramount importance in robotic exoskeletons working on the principle of internal forces. The typical misalignment between exoskeleton and anatomical joints results in uncomfortable interaction forces where both systems are attached to each other. Given the complex kinematics of most human anatomical joints, this problem is hard to avoid. The issue of compliant kinematics calls for bioinspired design of wearable robots and imposes a strong need for control of the human–robot physical interaction.

Exoskeletons are also characterized by a close cognitive interaction with the wearer. This cHRI is in most instances supported by the physical interface. By means of this cognitive interaction, the human commands and controls the robot, and in turn the robot includes the human in the control loop and provides information on the tasks, either by means of a force reflection mechanism or of some other kind of information.

1.4 Salient Issues in Exoskeletal Rehabilitation Robotics

The application of exoskeletons in rehabilitation scenarios encompasses multiple aspects that need to be carefully addressed. It is widely recognized that evolutionary biological processes lead to efficient behavioral and motor mechanisms. Evolution is a process whereby functional aspects of living creatures are optimized. This optimization process seeks the maximization of certain objective functions, e.g. manipulative dexterity in human hands and efficiency in terms of energy balance in performing a certain function. It is clear that the design of exoskeletal rehabilitation robots can benefit from biological models in a number of aspects like control, sensing and actuation. Likewise, exoskeletal rehabilitation robots can be used to understand and formalize models of biological motor control in humans. This concurrent view calls for a multidisciplinary approach to wearable robot development, which is where the concept of *Biomechatronics* comes in.

The term *Mechatronics* was coined in Japan in the mid 1970s and has been defined as the engineering discipline dealing with the study, analysis, design and implementation of hybrid systems comprising mechanical, electrical and control (intelligence) components or subsystems, [94]. Mechatronic systems closely linked to biological systems have been referred to as *bio–cybernetic systems* in the context of Electromyography (EMG) control of the full-body HAL–5 exoskeleton wearable robot system. The concept of *Biomechatronics* is not limited to bio–cybernetic systems.

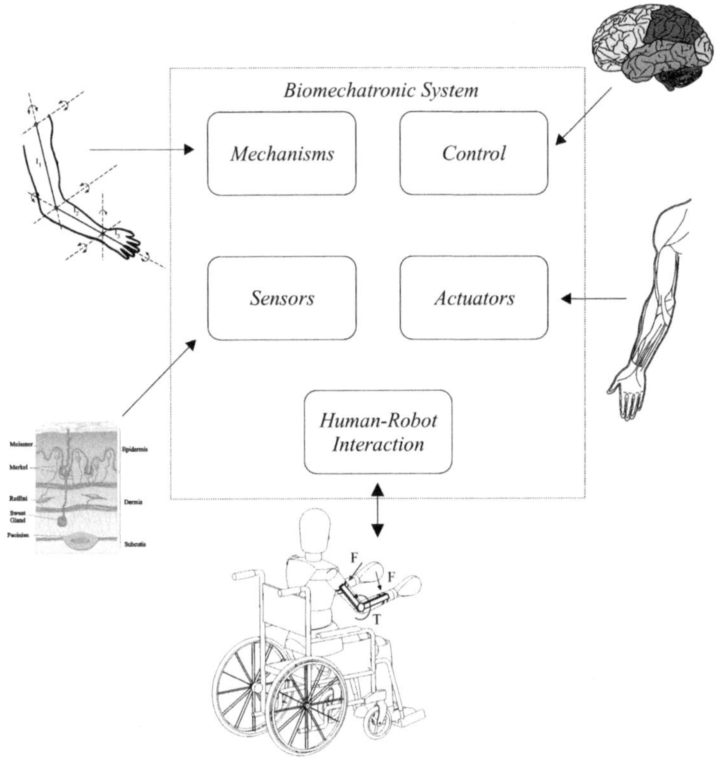

Fig. 1.4 Components in a biomechatronic system.

Biomechatronics can be analyzed by analogy to biological systems integrating a musculoskeletal apparatus with a nervous system, [27]. Following this analogy (see figure 1.4), biomechatronic systems integrate mechanisms, embedded control and Human–Machine Interaction (HMI), sensors, actuators and energy supply in such a way that each of these components, and the whole mechatronic system, is inspired by biological models. This book stresses the biomechatronic conception of wearable robots which are outlined in the following paragraphs.

1.4.1 Bioinspiration

Biomimetics is a relatively recent term coined in the 60s by Schmitt, [121, 138]. According to Webster's Dictionary, *biomimetics* is "the study of the formation, structure, or function of biologically produced substances and materials (as enzymes or silk) and biological mechanisms and processes (as protein synthesis or photosynthesis) especially for the purpose of synthesizing similar products by artificial mechanisms which mimic natural ones". However, the concept formalizes an idea already well established in western philosophy, for instance by ancient Greek philosophers like Aristotle, who stated: "If one way be better than another, that you may be sure is nature's way", or Democritus, who wrote: "We are pupils of the animals in the most important things: the spider for spinning and mending, the swallow for building, and the songsters, swan and nightingale, for singing, by way of imitation".

The understanding and modelling of biological systems has served as a source of inspiration in the design of different robotic systems. There are several reasons for a robot designer to study and model biological systems. One of the most important of these is the impressive performance of biological systems. Biological systems are able to deal with unpredictable situations; they can adapt, they can learn and they are robust to failure. It is therefore desirable to build artificial systems, e.g. wearable robots, with the same level of performance.

Moreover, physical or engineering models of biological systems (formalized mathematically) have proven very useful for understanding biological behavior. Models allow some manipulation of conditions that are very difficult to establish experimentally. Therefore, there is a mutual synergy between Engineering and Biology, see figure 1.5.

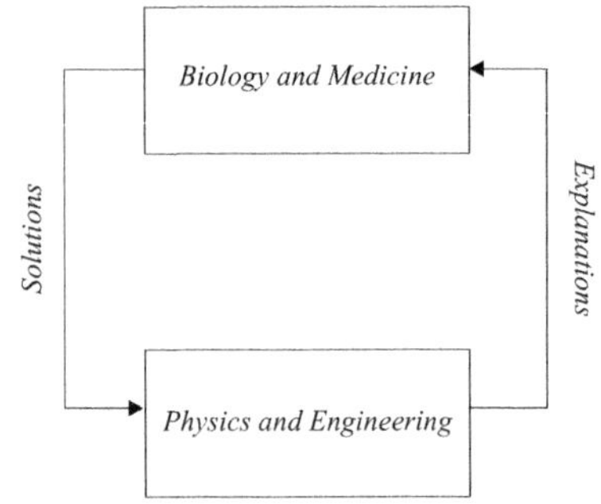

Fig. 1.5 Interaction of Biology and Medicine with Physics and Engineering. Biology can provide solutions for complex engineering problems, while mathematical models provide the most precise explanation for biological systems.

1.4.2 Mechanisms and Dynamic Models

This topic includes the particular kinematic and dynamic considerations of mapping robots onto human limb anatomy. It is interesting to note that, given certain reasonable assumptions, the methods used to study robots can also be used to analyze human kinematics and dynamics. For instance, one of the most common assumptions consists in modelling the human body as a chain of rigid links, where each segment has certain properties, like length or inertia, which approximate those of humans, see figure 1.6. These segments are linked by joints that imitate human ones in terms of degrees of freedom (DoFs) and ranges of motion (RoMs).

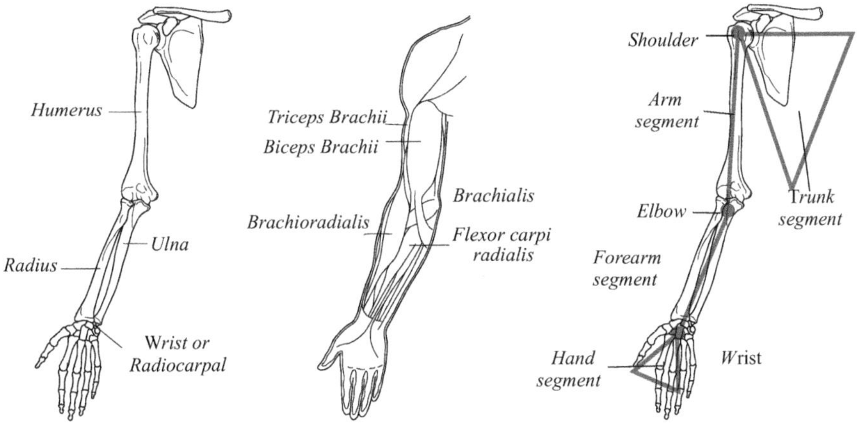

Fig. 1.6 Anatomy of the upper limb. Anterior view. (a) Bones (b) Muscles (c) Rigid-segment model.

This topic therefore encompasses both the mechanics of the robot and the human limbs. Along this book, the expression of the position and orientation of the robot is discussed in order to introduce the Denavit-Hartenberg convention algorithm, which makes a systematic method possible to describe robot position and orientation. The biomechanics of the upper and lower limbs are described briefly but in enough detail to show the derivation of the Denavit-Hartenberg parameters for the upper and lower limbs, this in the context of assessing tremor torque and power. The design aspects of wearable robotic exoskeletons are discussed in terms of the upper limb.

1.4.3 Physical HRI in the Context of Exoskeletal Robots

One important specific feature of Wearable Robotics is the intrinsic interaction between human and robot. This interaction, in its simplest manifestation, implies a physical coupling between the robot and the human, leading to the application of controlled forces between both actors. The actions of the two agents must be coordinated and adapted reciprocally since unexpected behavior of one of them during interaction can result in severe injuries. A classic example of physical interaction is exoskeleton-based functional compensation of human gait. Here, the robotic exoskeleton applies functional compensation by supporting human gait, i.e. by stabilizing the stance phase.

The fact that a human being is an integral part of the design is one of the most exciting and challenging aspects in the design of wearable robots. It imposes several constraints and requirements in the design of this kind of device. In this book, the term pHRI refers to Human-Robot physical Interaction and pHRi refers to Human-Robot physical Interface. In this book we will give details of the application a physical interaction between robot and human through a pHRi encompassing the robot structure and the human soft tissues in the context of tremor suppression. The authors consider that, without losing sight of the general picture, the design challenges for successful physical interaction are more illustrative in robots of this kind.

1.4.4 Cognitive HMI in the Context of Exoskeletal Robots

The symbiotic relationship between humans and robots transcends the boundaries of simple physical interaction. It involves smart sensors, actuators, algorithms and control strategies capable of gathering and decoding complex human expressions or physiological phenomena. Once this process is complete, robots use the information to adapt, learn and optimize their functions, or even to transmit back a response resulting from a cognitive process occurring within the robot.

New human-machine interfaces have recently been developed to support all the flow of information that a smart system needs in order to perform its function. Scientists consider this cognitive interaction fundamental. Thus we can find terms like Human-Machine Interface (HMI), Human-Computer Interface (HCI) and Brain-Computer Interface (BCI), all relating to this cognitive interaction. The search for a natural communication channel is a constant object of research, especially in the area of service robots, [104, 122]. In this book, the term cHRI stands for cognitive Human-Robot Interaction and HRi stands for cognitive Human-Robot Interface.

New trends in cHRI are moving in the direction of sourcing the information directly from the human cognitive processes involved in the normal execution of tasks. These are called natural interfaces. The rationale for this approach comes from, [124]:

- Biological reasons. cHRI systems seek to take advantage of the natural control mechanisms fully optimized in humans. Moreover, a lot of information is lost in the translation of biologically executed tasks into discrete events, e.g. natural movements or gestures into buttons or joysticks.
- Practical reasons. Delays are introduced when natural cognitive processes are encoded into an imposed sequence of tasks. In addition, a training phase is needed to teach the user to generate these non-natural commands or to map a cognitive process into a new set of outputs. Both factors, the delays and the mapping, can induce fatigue in the user, both at a musculo-skeletal level and at a

mental level. These factors can be obviated if the natural outputs of a cognitive process are used for cHRI.
- Rehabilitation. One of the main applications of exoskeletons, and in particular the one that we focus on in this book, is rehabilitation. Interacting directly with the phenomena involved in the cognitive process is a means to excite them and assess the evolution of the rehabilitation therapy.

The design of a cHRI depends on the kind of information to be transmitted. Figure 1.7 depicts the cHRI concepts. There are unidirectional interfaces to control robots, bidirectional interfaces, or closed loop interaction, e.g. in haptic applications. Unidirectional interfaces are defined as interfaces where the subject has no information about the state of the system immediately after a command is sent. Bidirectional interfaces provide feedback immediately after the command is sent by the user. Closed loop systems are defined as continuous symbiotic interaction between user and robotic system. The closed loop interaction can enhance the user's situation awareness, increasing efficiency and achieving control in a way that is more natural to the user, [122].

The role of the different components of a cHRI and the interaction environment are also depicted in figure 1.7. The role of the sensors is to measure the human-related phenomena, while the actuators have to transmit the robotic cognitive information to the user to complement his sensory information about the task.

The interaction environment is a key issue for natural cHRIs. The aim of modern interfaces is to avoid saturating the biological cognitive channels, and therefore

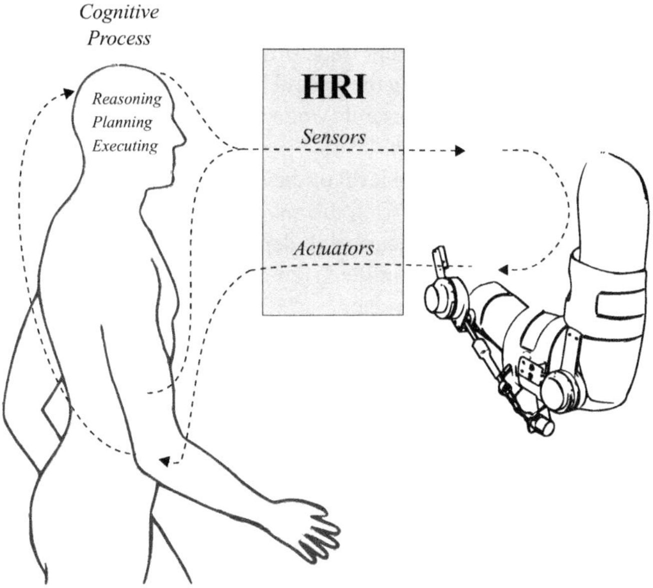

Fig. 1.7 The information flow from user reasoning to final execution of the action, showing the signals acquired though the information pathway.

new ones are being explored. Figure 1.7 shows three levels of interaction: one related to reasoning and planning, one related to muscle activity and one related to the wearer's motion. The planning level interaction can be accomplished by monitoring brain activity using different techniques, e.g. electroencephalography or brain implanted electrodes. The muscle activity level uses muscle electrical activity, that is EMG, to command the devices. This activity can be acquired even without limb movement. The movement-related level of interaction uses kinematic and kinetic information from the subject as control inputs. Multimodal approaches propose diversified use of these channels in order to gather more realistic and robust information and to gain a better understanding of the phenomena by means of data fusion techniques.

1.4.5 Sensors, Actuators and Supporting Technologies

The interface between human and robot can exchange signals in order to drive an action, provide feedback for human motor control, and monitor the status of the HRI and its surroundings. *Wearability* within an application imposes a number of particular requirements on sensor, actuator and energy storage technologies. A comparative analysis of the state-of-the-art technologies is needed for each category, providing an overview of the current achievements in technology development.

When defining reliable sensors for a wearable application it may be useful to analyze a wide range of candidate measurement devices. Measurement requirements for a system may consider or combine accurate tracking of movement or force, quantification of the status of the HR interface, acquisition of a physiological signal for feedback, etc. In order to equip a wearable robot with a measurement system, the designer must unavoidably accept trade offs between functional versatility and simplicity of implementation. Using the natural body as a sensing mechanism can be an elegant solution to enhance the usability of a WR and also to overcome particular challenges imposed by applications.

Actuators may be required at the level of the human joints or limbs, to respond to signals from the human body and from the environment. Whether a given actuator technology is considered for integration will depend on the type of physical interaction with the limb that is required in the given range of applications, e.g. damping, modulation of resistance, powering, etc.

1.5 Scope of the Book

The main objective of the study presented in this book is to investigate the application of robotic exoskeletons for active upper limb tremor suppression. This work was developed in the framework of the European Project DRIFTS (EU QoL QLK6-CT-2002-00536). This project was launched on 2002 to validate the concept of tremor suppression through wearable orthotic devices. The methodology used to reach this objective was based on a detailed review of research work in the generic area of tremor management during the last decades. In particular special focus has been put on the systems approach and thus a specific section on modelling has been included. Aspects related to experimental protocol and tremor pattern identification are reviewed in detail with the aim of drawing a practical guideline when compensatory technology has to be developed. This review identified the gaps in the literature of orthotic tremor management and defined the base for the development of the work presented in this book. In summary, the mains gaps identified were:

- The lack of research focused on orthotic pathologic tremor suppression.
- There is an absence of studies in the literature centered in the analysis of the tremor behavior in each articulation of the upper limb.
- The development of algorithms with low computation cost able to distinguish in real-time tremor from voluntary motion is required.
- The non-existence of biomechanical studies related to upper limb tremor.
- There is a clear need in the rehabilitation area of ambulatory devices able to apply dynamic forces to the upper limb.
- The absence of control strategies for selective tremor suppression: the orthosis should minimize involuntary limb movements while preserving the voluntary limb motion.

The work presented in this book tried to fill these gaps. The main contributions to the literature of this work are summarized in the following points:

- The development of a sensor solution based on gyroscopes for the estimation of tremor in the different joint of the upper limb.
- The definition of an interesting novel method (Empirical Mode Decomposition: EMD) to analyze tremor recordings with superimposed voluntary or other involuntary movement components. It is shown convincingly that this automatized method performs as well as 'manual' filtering to separate the different components. A second method, the Hilbert Spectrum (HS) is then introduced to analyze the frequency contents of the different components over time. All in all the methods and their value in tremor analysis are well documented warranting further trials applying these methods in tremor analysis.
- The analysis of tremor behavior at different joints of the upper limb.
- The development of an algorithm able to estimate tremor in real-time and with a low computational cost.
- The definition and the development of an upper limb exoskeleton able to apply dynamics forces between segments of the upper limb.
- The definition of novel control strategies for tremor suppression without loading the voluntary motion.
- The presentation of a clinical evaluation of the exoskeleton for tremor suppression. It performance was assessed in 10 patients suffering from different tremors pathologies.
- The definition of the limitations, requirements and milestones in the robotic field so that the exoskeletons for ambulatory tremor suppression overcome the status of laboratory robots.

The book is organized in four thematic chapters (chapters 2 through 5) dealing with all relevant aspects to tremor management and control of wearable robots in close cooperation with human actors. At the end of the book, chapter 6 summarizes the most relevant topics discussed in the book and briefly presents an outlook of future development and likely research avenues. Figure 1.8 illustrate the structure of the book and the relations amongst chapters. The following paragraphs briefly summarize the scope of the book and of each chapter.

Chapter 2 presents a detailed review on the stat-of-th-art of tremor. Users groups are identified according to different characteristics of the pathology (rest, postural

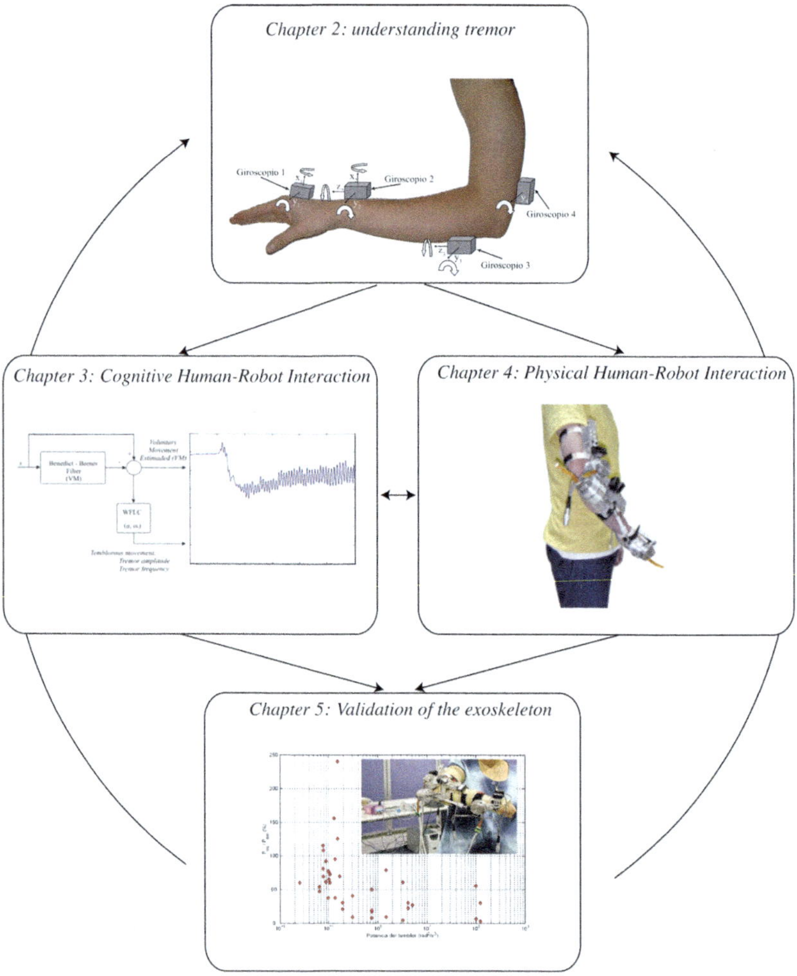

Fig. 1.8 Structure of the book to stress the de development and validation of an upper limb exoskeleton for tremor suppression. Notice that it illustrates the learning loop, since the validation of the exoskeleton developed provided new knowledge on tremor.

and kinetic tremor). The main characteristics of tremor according to the pathology are given. Based on this extensive review, it was identified that most of the research on tremor movements are focused on studying tremor at distal parts of the upper limb. There is a lack of studies centered in the analysis of the tremor behavior in each articulation of the upper limb. Moreover, there is no consensus in the optimal way to objectively measure tremor in the upper limb. In this chapter the authors proposed a new approach for tremor assessment based on gyroscopes. Moreover, a novel tool for the analysis of tremor time series is introduced. The main advantage of this technique it that it allows an automatic estimate of the tremorous movement in the different pathologies considered in this study. The application of this technique introduces new attributes to the tremorous signal such as instantaneous amplitude, instantaneous phase and instantaneous frequency. Based on this new methodology, a study of tremor behavior at joint level was performed and is presented in this chapter. This study brings new knowledge to the tremor field and pave the way for the development of upper limb exoskeletons for tremor suppression.

Chapter 3 addresses the cognitive HumanRobot interaction (cHRI) between the upper-limb exoskeleton and the human. This CHRI is based on the information provided by gyroscopes and force sensors, which measures the movement at each joint of the upper limb and the interaction force between the robot and the human, respectively. The algorithm presented is able to estimate in real-time tremor amplitude and frequency based on IMU information. Quantification of instantaneous tremor parameters plays an important role in robotics based tremor management techniques in order to efficiently exploit the possibilities of biomechanical loading without affecting the voluntary movement of the patient. The algorithm developed presents the following advantages for its application in ambulatory devices for tremor suppression: a) Estimate the voluntary movement, b) Estimate the tremorous movement, c) The delay introduced for the estimation is 1 ms and the convergence time is always smaller than 2 s, d) Estimate both the amplitude and the frequency of the tremorous movement, e) Presents a low computation cost.

Chapter 4 is focused on the study of the dynamics of the man-machine physical interaction. This physical interaction is performed by the robotic exoskeleton WOTAS (Wearable Orthosis for Tremor Assessment and Suppression) that provides a means of testing and validating ungrounded control strategies for orthotic tremor suppression. It describes in detail the general concept for WOTAS, outlining the special features of the design and selection of system components. Two control strategies developed for tremor suppression with exoskeletons are described. These two strategies are based on biomechanical loading and notch filtering the tremor through the application of internal forces.

Chapter 5 is dedicated to the validation and discussion of the different aspect related to the issues presented in the book. This chapter included the definition of the experimental protocol defined for the validation of the exoskeleton developed, the selection fo patients suffering from different pathologies that induces tremor (Essential tremor, Parkinson Disease and Cerebellar tremor), and the definition of the metrics used to evaluate the performance of the exoskeleton in the suppression of tremor. Results from experiments using the two strategies defined in the previous chapter on patients with tremor are summarized. Finally, results from clinical trials are presented, which indicate the feasibility of ambulatory mechanical suppression of tremor.

Finally, the conclusions and future work of this study are described in *Chapter 6*. This chapter introduces the new research lines opened by the work described in this book.

Chapter 2
Pathological Tremor Management

A great deal of effort has been devoted in the past decades in the generic area of tremor management. Specific topics of modelling for objective classification of pathological tremor out of kinematics and physiological data, compensatory technologies and evaluation rating tools are just a few examples of application field. This chapter introduces a comprehensive review of research work in this generic field during the last decades. In particular special focus has been put on the systems approach and thus a specific section on modelling has been included. Aspects related to experimental protocol and tremor pattern identification are reviewed in detail with the aim of drawing a practical guideline when compensatory technology has to be developed. The current status on ambulatory and non-ambulatory tremor reduction technologies is given in the section devoted to tremor management. At the end, we finish our discussion with those aspects related to tremor evaluation.

2.1 Introduction

Tremor is a rhythmic, involuntary muscular contraction characterised by oscillations (to-and-from movements) of a part of the body, [7]. Although the most common types of tremor were subject to numerous studies, their mechanisms and origins are still unknown. The most common of all involuntary movements, tremor can affect various body parts such as the hands, head, facial structures, tongue, trunk, and legs; most tremors, however, occur in the hands. Tremor often accompanies neurological disorders associated with aging. Although the disorder is not life-threatening, it can be responsible for functional disability and social embarrassment, [33].

There are many types of tremor and several ways in which tremor is classified, [37]. The most common classification is by behavioural context or position, [33]. There are five categories of tremor within this classification: resting, postural, kinetic, task-specific, and hysterical. It is accepted that the majority of the affected patients have either Parkinson disease or Essential tremor and that the most incapacitating are essential tremor, tremor due to Parkinson disease and cerebellar tremor.

E. Rocon and J.L. Pons: Exoskeletons in Rehabilitation Robotics, STAR 69, pp. 21–51.
springerlink.com

Resting or static tremor occurs when the muscle is at rest, for example when the hands are lying on the lap. This type of tremor is often seen in patients with Parkinson's disease. Postural tremor occurs when a patient attempts to maintain posture, such as holding the hands outstretched. Postural tremors include physiological tremor, essential tremor, tremor with basal ganglia disease (also seen in patients with Parkinson's disease), cerebellar postural tremor, tremor with peripheral neuropathy, post-traumatic tremor, and alcoholic tremor. Kinetic tremor occurs during purposeful movement, for example during finger-to-nose testing. Task-specific tremor appears when performing goal-oriented tasks such as handwriting, speaking, or standing. This group consists of primary writing tremor, vocal tremor, and orthostatic tremor.

Tremor is a disorder that is not life-threatening, but it can be responsible for functional disability and social embarrassment. More than 65% of the population with upper limb tremor present serious difficulties performing daily living activities, [46]. In many cases, tremor intensities are very large, causing total disability to the affected person.

The effect of tremor on the patient depends on the clinical manifestation. In general it can be said that the more goal-directed movements are distorted by tremor, the more severe the difficulty in performing daily activities. On the other hand, rest tremor is seen by the patients as a cause for social exclusion.

2.2 Tremor Manifestations

There are many types of tremor and several ways in which tremor is classified. The most common classification is by behavioural context or position, [37]. There are five categories of tremor within this classification: resting, postural, kinetic, task-specific, and hysterical. Resting or static tremor occurs when the muscle is at rest, for example when the hands are lying on the lap. This type of tremor is often seen in patients with Parkinson's disease. Postural tremor occurs when a patient attempts to maintain posture, such as holding the hands outstretched. Postural tremors include physiological tremor, essential tremor, tremor with basal ganglia disease (also seen in patients with Parkinson's disease), cerebellar postural tremor, tremor with peripheral neuropathy, post-traumatic tremor, and alcoholic tremor. Kinetic or intention (action) tremor occurs during purposeful movement, for example during finger-to-nose testing. Task-specific tremor appears when performing goal-oriented tasks such as handwriting, speaking, or standing. This group consists of primary writing tremor, vocal tremor, and orthostatic tremor. Hysterical tremor (also called psychogenic tremor) occurs in both older and younger patients. The key feature of this tremor is that it dramatically lessens or disappears when the patient is distracted.

The aetiology of tremor is diverse and different activation circumstances can be present, [33]. Table 2.1 summarises this situation.

Table 2.1 Aetiology of tremor

Tremor type	Affected limbs	Frequency pattern	Mechanical characteristics	Remarks
Essential (postural and kinetic)	Abduction-adduction of fingers; Flexion-extension of wrist; Pronation-supination of forearm	5 to 8 Hz (Jain et al.), 4 to 12 Hz (Cooper et al.), 3 to 11 Hz (Elble) Invariant upon mechanical loading (< 1 Hz)	Mean tremor amplitude of $13\frac{rad}{s2}$ (Elble); Amplitude increases with aging or progression; Power estimation: 1.7 W (wrist $\pm 30^o$ @ 3 Hz).	Frequency decrease with time (0.06-0.08 Hz yearly); Rhythmic bursts in EMG Symmetric.
Parkinsonian (rest)	Flexion-extension of fingers, i.e. "pill-rolling movement″ Flexion-extension of wrist Pronation-supination of forearm	3 to 6 Hz	Presence of tremor at rest, muscular stiffness, acknesia and postural instability. It affects distal parts of the body but propagates to proximal parts with the evolution of the disease	Suppression under voluntary muscle contraction. Originally distal, extending to proximal body parts.
Cerebellar (intention and kinetic)	Proximal muscles are more commonly affected. Flexion-extension of wrist	2 to 4 Hz Invariant upon external loading	Muscle torque driving the oscillation independent of external loads. Tremor amplitude up to $\pm 30^o$	Bilateral and symmetric Synchronous EMG in flexors, extensors or both. EMG, acceleration and torque are stationary.

2.3 Tremor Patterns

As described above, tremor denotes an involuntary oscillation of limbs of the body. A number of works tried to model tremor but so far no tremor is understood completely, [44, 64, 108]. Human physiological tremor is surrounded by a long history of controversy and general interest, [33]. Most of the interest is based on the beliefs that tremor offers some clue to the mechanisms of neuromuscular control in man and the clarification of physiological tremor will help to elucidate the origins of many pathological action tremors.

Pioneered in the work of Lippold, [76], various experiments were performed to clarify the effect of reflex mechanisms on physiological tremor. According to Lippold the reflex mechanisms which stabilise a limb during maintained posture may also be responsible for physiological tremor. This possibility arises from the fact that there are substantial delays in the feedback from muscle so that at certain frequencies (8-12Hz) the feedback is sufficiently delayed so that it adds to the next phase of the movement, rather than resisting the phase that produced it.

Based on the Lippold work, Stein and Oguztreli, [125] introduced a deterministic model concerning the properties of muscles and the sensory feedback pathways from muscles in order to evaluate the tremor sources. Stein used a stochastic feedback system which applies a signoidal nonlinearity describing the activation function of the motoneurons. According to Stein, damped oscillations can arise in the absence of sensory feedback due to interaction of a muscle with inertial loads. Stein is one of the researchers that performed an experiment to clarify the effect of reflex mechanisms on physiological tremor.

Other studies address the problem of determining the excitation sources of normal tremor. In particular, Stiles focuses on determining to what extent mechanical and neural factors are involved in the excitation of physiological tremor, [126]. In 1998, Timmer used cross-spectral analysis to study the role of reflexes in physiological tremor, [129]. Cross-spectral analysis has the advantage of not perturbing the system, i.e. the stimulus for the reflexes is the tremor itself.

Timmer is one of the researchers that pay more attention to modelling tremor. Initially, the standard methods of stochastic and deterministic time series analysis were used to analyse data of various physiological and pathological forms of tremor. Timmer et al. had shown that the physiological tremor can be described as a linear stochastic process whereas pathological forms of tremor represent non-linear processes, [128] . He used a stochastic feedback system which applies a sigmoidal nonlinearity describing the activation function of the motoneurons that was introduced by Stein. In this work Timmer gives evidence for the contribution of the reflexes to the tremor. However, there is no evidence in the data that reflex loops primarily cause the tremor. Reflex loops alter the frequency, relaxation time, and amplitude of existing oscillation to some degree. Therefore, Timmer supports that the primary cause of physiological tremor is the resonant behaviour of the hand and a synchronised EMG activity that is either generated centrally or due to the recruitment strategy of motoneurons. Other researchers tried to model the behaviour of a limb affected by tremor. In 1973, Randall suggested linear stochastic autoregressive processes to model the tremor data, [103]. Randall used digitised samples of hand acceleration in order to construct a stochastic time series model for hand tremor. This study showed that of the part of tremor variance which can be explained by the difference equation, the major portion was explained by a second-order difference equation having a natural frequency of about 10 Hz (ω_n) and a damping ratio of about 0,10 (ξ). The unexplained part was essentially white noise and would be the random noise driving the frequency-selective part, as illustrated by the following second-order difference equation:

$$y''(t) + 2\xi\,\omega_n y'(t) + \omega_n y(t) = 0 \qquad (2.1)$$

The different manifestations of normal or physiological tremor have been extensively analysed during the past decades. In particular, Elble, [33], carefully examined the relation between hand tremor and the 8-12 Hz component of finger tremor, that is the range of frequency that received the most attention, largely because of the work of Lippold, [76]. Previous work, [128], showed that physiological tremor can be regarded as a linear stochastic process consistent with the interpretation of a mechanical system of the hand as a damped linear oscillator driven by a uncorrelated firing of motoneurons. These results suggest that features, especially of nonlinear dynamics, may lead to a good classification of the different kinds of tremor.

Pathological tremor exhibits a nonlinear oscillation that is not strictly periodic. Timmer et al, [130], investigated whether the deviation from periodicity is due to nonlinear deterministic chaotic dynamics or due to nonlinear stochastic dynamics. To do so, Timmer applied various methods from linear and nonlinear time series analysis to tremor time series. The results of the different methods suggest that the considered types of pathological tremors represent nonlinear stochastic second order processes. Finally, Timmer investigated whether two earlier proposed features capturing nonlinear effects in the time series allow for discrimination between two pathological forms of tremor for a much larger sample of time series than previously investigated.

According to Timmer, tremor time series span a large range of different behaviours. The physiological tremor of healthy subjects represents a linear second order stochastic process driven by white noise originating from uncorrelated firing of motoneurons, [129]. The enhanced physiological tremor can either be described by a stochastic linear second order process driven by colored noise or non-linear stochastic delay differential equation depending on the degree of the contribution of a central pacemaker or of reflexes, [130]. Timmer also support that pathological tremor like essential, Parkinson, and Kinetic tremor exhibit a non-linear oscillation. The oscillation is not strictly periodic. Timmer is researching the possible reasons for the deviation from a strictly periodic, limit cycle type of dynamics. According to Timmer, the oscillation of the pathological tremors is best described by a non-linear stochastic second order process. This affirmation contradict the suggestion of Gresty et al., [48], that the variability observed in the considered pathological tremors should be interpreted as caused by frequency and/or amplitude modulated harmonic oscillators.

The different manifestations of normal or physiologic tremor have been extensively analysed during the past decades. As described below, there is sufficient evidence that supports the fact that oscillating limbs behave as second order biomechanical systems relating input muscle torque to output limb position. Adelstein in his thesis gives evidence of this second order behaviour, [1]:

- The frequency of the oscillating peaks in subjects with normal physiologic tremor is inversely related to the square root of the lumped sum of the inertia of the body part and the externally added mass.
- The effect of varying the limb stiffness (of the forearm) results in a frequency change directly related to the equivalent stiffness.

From the point of view of the applicability of tremor-suppression exoskeletons, this book is mainly interested in Essential, Parkinsonian and kinetic tremor. Following the characteristic patterns of these forms of tremor are reviewed.

2.3.1 Essential Tremor

This is the most common form of pathological tremor. Moreover, it is the pathology with more incidence among all the movement disorders, [7]. More than five million of americans citizens, the majority older than 60 years, are affected by Essential tremor. Essential tremor may begin in childhood but it is usually seen later in life and persists through adulthood. The mean age at onset is between 35 and 45 years and it is slowly progressive, tremor frequency declines and amplitude increases. When severe it can be disabling and result in difficulty in writing and in handling tools or eating utensils. Up to 25% of the patients with this condition retire or change jobs as a result of tremor.

Essential tremor (ET) is defined by a bilateral postural tremor involving the upper limbs, [70]. Essential tremor is typically symmetric affecting both upper limbs in particular the hands and forearms, [7]. Koller states that it appears most frequently in the hands, being abduction-adduction of fingers and flexion-extension of wrist typically affected, [70]. In some cases it also affects pronation-supination of the forearm.

A kinetic tremor, increasing in amplitude when the limb approaches a target, is often observed, and a head tremor may be associated. ET is postural and kinetic and a rest component is rarely found and always in the most advanced cases. It is always accompanied by a rhythmic entrainment of the motor units discharge that forces the affected body into oscillation. This results in rhythmic bursts in the EMG of the involved muscles. Mechanical loading has little effect on the frequency characteristics of Essential tremor, typically <1 Hz, [35]. The frequency band of Essential tremor differs according to the reporting author, while Jain, [64], gives relatively narrow frequency band of 5 to 8 Hz, Elble gives 3 to 11 Hz, [35].

ET, a heterogeneous disorder, is the most common movement disorder in adults, with an estimated prevalence of 4% (2-3). Possible non-motor manifestations of ET, such as mood fluctuations or personality disorders, require further work prior stating that they could share similar mechanisms with motor symptoms, [77]. Symptoms typically are progressive and disabling. The link between ET and Parkinsons disease is often a matter of debate, [78].

The mechanism of ET remains to be elucidated, [37]. According to animal models of ET, an abnormal olivo-cerebellar activity would result in enhanced oscillatory activity in the cerebellum and its target nuclei in the thalamic circuits. However, recordings of neurons in human are not consistent with the theory of continuous olivo-cerebellar driving of the motor cortex via thalamic connections. ET might be induced by networks enabling tremor-related activity during voluntary movement and by enhanced access of sensory feedback. To the light of the role of the cerebellum in sensorimotor processing, a pathological coupling between sensory inputs and motor output may be considered, [83]. There is evidence from behavioural studies and imaging techniques that the cerebellar circuit is a plausible site for the genesis of ET. The clinical similarities between symptoms of ET and the symptoms in classical cerebellar disorders is obvious, [70].

For a given patient the Essential tremor frequency decreases at a rate of 0.06 to 0.08 Hz yearly, however, Elble found that tremor frequency is a function of age but not of duration illness. The age, a, and frequency, f, of unit motor entrainment in the forearms of these patients show the following linear relationship:

$$f = -0.077a + 11.4 \tag{2.2}$$

Following with the characterisation of the essential tremor, Elble found a logarithmic relationship between tremor amplitude, A, frequency, f, and the amplitude of the EMG, v:

$$log(A) = \alpha log(f) + \beta log(v) \tag{2.3}$$

Little figures were found in the literature about Essential tremor amplitude. Just Elble reports that the mean value of the tremor acceleration amplitude was $2\frac{m}{s^2}$. This figure was obtained with the forearm pronated and supported in such a way that only motion about the wrist was allowed.

In our literature review we have only found estimations on the power for Essential tremor due to Kotovsky, [71]. They assume the tremor to follow a sinusoidal pattern with a frequency of 3 Hz and tremor amplitude of 30° (severe tremor). They adopt a worst case assumption to establish an upper bound on the power that should be dissipated by an active orthosis. They assume that: (1) the muscle torque exciting the tremor is not reduced with the addition of the orthosis, (2) all the muscle torque in the presence of the orthosis must be dissipated by the orthosis itself (none is applied to the elastic and innertial elemnets). Under these conditions the power to be dissipated results in 1.7 W.

2.3.2 *Parkinsonian tremor*

Parkinson disease is a chronic, slowly progressive degenerative disorder of the central nervous system that was first described by James Parkinson in 1817 as "paralysis agitans. It is characterized by the presence of a resting tremor, rigidity, akinesia, and postural instability. The principal pathology of Parkinsons disease is loss of dopaminergic cells in the substantia nigra pars compacta, and this abnormality is responsible for most, if not all, of the motor abnormalities, including tremor. However, the source of oscillation in parkinsonian tremor is still uncertain.

As reported by Koller, [70], men and women appear to be affected equally. Parkinson disease ranks behind cerebrovascular diseases and arthritis as the third most common chronic disease of the late adulthood, [35]. The incidence increase with age, with the peak onset between the sixth and eight decades. Familial occurrences are seen, but the lack of concordance in twins indicates the absence of a strong genetic factor, [64]. It affects 1% of the population over the age of 50 in US with an estimated incidence of 40,000 new cases per year, [35]. Other authors report slightly lower prevalence figures. In particular Deuschl, [30], gives an overall prevalence of 110 cases per 100,000.

Parkinsonian tremor is a rest tremor affecting flexion-extension of the thumb against the index finger, flexion-extension of the wrist and pronation-supination of the forearm. The voluntary muscle contraction typically suppresses Parkinsonian rest tremor, but it is generally followed by a mild to moderate action tremor. Jain, [64], in his research, discovered that in Parkinson disease, all aspects of movement are affected, including initiation, execution, and the ability to halt a movement once it has begun. In the majority of patients, Parkinson disease develops insidiously and progresses slowly. There are often long periods during which the progression is so slow that it appears to be in a partial remission.

As reported by Elble, in many patients the rest tremor persists during posture and movement, typically with lower amplitude, but with no change in frequency or EMG characteristics. In other patients the action tremor has slightly higher frequency, [35]. The frequency band of this tremor ranges from 3 to 6 Hz, as reported by Jain, [64]. Cooper supports that Parkinson tremor is commonly associated with a 4-6 Hz rest tremor that is often asymmetric, [24]. It is originally distal and extends to more proximal body parts as Parkinson progresses.

2.3.3 *Cerebellar tremor*

The most common type of cerebellar tremor is kinetic, or goal directed. Gordon Holmes used the term intention tremor to describe the tremors that are observed in patients with cerebellar lesions, [60]. According to Jain, a kinetic tremor is seen in cerebellar dysfunction as an oscillatory ataxia of proximal muscles, [64]. It is a jerky, arrhythmic interruption of the normal progression of voluntary motion and becomes more pronounced as greater precision is demanded. Once the target is reached, the tremor ceases. The frequency of the tremor varies from 3 to 5 Hz. Hallet in his work remarked that multiple sclerosis is the most common cause of the cerebellar postural tremor, [49]. Other causes of this tremor include tumors, strokes, and brain traumas, as well as neural degeneration in the cerebellum.

During examination, a cerebellar tremor increases in severity as the extremity approaches its target. Other signs of cerebellar pathology, such as abnormalities of gait, speech and ocular movements, and the ability to perform rapidly alternating movements, may be present and may help to confirm the diagnosis of cerebellar tremor. Many medications have been tried with little or no benefit in the treatment of cerebellar tremor. This is not surprising, given the pathophysiological complexity of the oscillating transcortical and transcerebellar pathways, [35, 37]. The added inertia of wrist weights attenuates cerebellar tremor and is useful in some patients, [71]. In general a lack of figures on prevalence of tremor following cerebellar trauma is observed in the literature.

The most common form of cerebellar tremor is an intention tremor of frequency lower than 5 Hz. The tremor is typically bilateral and symmetric when caused by a degenerative or toxic disorder, [24]. The most thorough study on the pattern of intention tremor is due to Adelstein, [1]. It was conducted on a group of patients exhibiting intention tremor of diverse etiological origins. It was conducted under two conditions, namely free wrist rotation and complete isometric restrain. The tremor characteristics as reported by Adelstein are as follows:

- The frequency band ranges from 2 to 4 Hz.
- The frequency band is independent of external loading both under additional viscous damping and isometric constrain
- The EMG shows synchronous bursts in flexors, extensors or both simultaneously.
- Under isometric constrain tremor activity is found in the measured torque.
- All the measured signals (EMG, acceleration and torque) are stationary.
- The comparison of torque densities associated to the isometric tremor spectral peaks and estimated from free oscillation trials indicated that the torque driving the oscillating tremor is independent of the magnitude of externally applied loads.

Other works, see Manyam [82], show that the kinetic cerebellar tremor is characterised by oscillation of variable amplitude and perpendicular to the direction of movement. Proximal muscles are most commonly affected, and the tremor amplitude can reach up to 30 degrees. According to Manyam the frequency of cerebellar kinetic is commonly described as being 3-5 Hz, but studies have shown that the frequency of cerebellar is inversely proportional to limb inertia, resulting in frequency being dependent on the part of the affect limb. In the upper extremities, kinetic tremor has a frequency of 3-8 Hz, and in the lower extremities is usually 3 Hz. The truncal tremor usually has a frequency of 2-4 Hz.

2.4 Tremor Characterization at Joint Level

A number of papers discuss the quantification of tremor. Quantification of tremor is of clinical interest as an aid to diagnosis and to evaluate objectively the effect of treatment. Hand writing and drawing patterns are often used to examine tremor. Recording such patterns using a digitising tablet has been introduced as one way to provide precise quantification. Most of these studies are focused on assessing tremor at distar part of the arm, since tremor is more disabling and visible at this level. There is an absense of studies in the literature centred in the analyis of tremor behaviour in each joint of the upper limb. The analysis of tremor at joint level is crucial for the design of robotic solutions for tremor suppression, for instance the selection of appropiate actuator technology to be used by a power exoskeleton. This section will be focused on studying tremor behaviour at joint level.

Clinical classification of tremor is based on the body parts involved, position of maximum activation, morphology, and frequency. From the point of view of tremor quantification, the two most important factors are the frequency and the amplitude. Frequency of tremor has been often given much importance and is used in classification, [35]. Amplitude of tremor is easily quantifiable and is classified as middle, moderate, and severe on various rating scales. It is important to show up that the amplitude of tremor in patients with the same disease may vary and can be increased by physical and emotional stress.

Gao used dynamical systems theory in order to discriminate between essential and Parkinsonian tremors and has shown that pathological tremors can be characterised as diffusional processes, [44]. He concluded that the quantities that might be able to discriminate among different pathological tremors should be purely of dynamical origin, since quantities that are purely of dynamical origin characterise more the similarities than the differences among different pathological tremors, as summarized in his studies. Gao used a non-dynamical quantity $\frac{L}{T}$, which is the ratio between the embedding delay time and the mean oscillation period, and concluded that it is a much more promising figure of merit in discriminating between essential and Parkinsonian tremors. On the other hand, Timmer showed that these kinds of tremor can be characterised as different non-linear processes.

According to Elble, tremor is well suited to spectral analysis, the most popular method of tremor quantification, because of its oscillatory characteristic, [33]. The idea is to calculate a power spectral density function indicating the signal power at different frequencies across the spectrum. The dominant frequency of tremor is evident in the form of a peak in the power spectral density, while the average tremor amplitude can be determined from the area under the peak. Riviere used a computational method, the weighted frequency Fourier linear combiner (WFLC), for quantification of tremor, [107]. This technique rapidly determines the frequency and amplitude of tremor by adjusting its filter weights according to a gradient search method. It provides continual tracking of frequency and amplitude modulations over the course of a test.

Others researches, i.e. Beuter and Edwards, [31, 32], focused their studies on the use of time and frequency domain characteristics to discriminate among the various types of tremor. Their studies showed that time domain and frequency domain characteristics can enhance the diagnostic power of tremor and could eventually be used by clinicians and epidemiologists to detect subclinical changes in tremor.

The detection and quantification of tremor are of clinical interest for diagnosis of neurological disorders and objective evaluation of their treatment, [108, 128, 129]. Methods based on the Fourier transform (FT) are commonly employed for this purpose, specially because of the similarity between the tremor to a sine wave, [34]. Some inherent drawbacks of techniques based on the FT are pointed out in [3, 4]. First, the signal is *linearly* decomposed as combination of sines and cosines.

Secondly, the compromise between time and frequency resolution of methods based on the FT may not highlight the presence of local oscillations in the signal which can have important physical meaning.

Recently, a novel technique for analysis of nonlinear and nonstationary time-series, was successfully applied to investigations of seismological and biological signals. This technique was first introduced in [61], and it is formed by two complementary tools, which are called Empirical Mode Decomposition (EMD) and Hilbert spectrum (HS). The EMD decomposes any arbitrary time-series into a set of components designated as intrinsic mode functions (IMFs). The main aim of the EMD is to iteratively identify distinct time-scales (or frequency bandwidths) from the data themselves that may have a physical meaning, e.g. IMFs may be related to biological phenomena. The existence of such a meaning is not guaranteed and an important issue in any practical investigation applying this technique is to define or identify it.

Once IMFs are extracted from the signal it is possible to analyze how their energy evolves as a function of time and frequency on the Hilbert spectrum (HS). In contrast to the spectrogram (based on the FT) the HS is a windowing independent time-frequency representation that may provide enough resolution in the signal analysis for detection of events often obscured in a conventional analysis. Examples showing the gain in resolution provided by the HS when compared to the spectrogram and scalogram (wavelets) are given in [61].

This section introduces the application of the EMD and HS as an alternative tool to the study of tremor. First we show that in this context, IMFs have a physical meaning, that is, single IMFs may represent either voluntary or involuntary movement activity of patients. The identification of such a physical meaning for IMFs is relevant because it shows that the method can automatically detect tremor. Note that the automatic detection of tremor is an important stage in systems that aim to control limb oscillations, and also in biofeedback studies. Secondly, it was shown that other physiological events that normally accompany the tremor, e.g. spasms, may also be identified in some IMFs.

In a further analysis, Hilbert spectrum was used to visualize how the energy of IMFs vary as a function of time and frequency. This study showed that the energy of voluntary and involuntary movement activity could be well distinguished on the HS. This result may be useful for investigations that aim to classify distinct neurological disorders, as the precise characterization of the energy of abnormal oscillations in limbs is a crucial stage in these studies. Results are based on an extensive analysis of signals collected from 31 subjects suffering from distinct neurological disorders and executing different types of movements or tasks.

2.4.1 Measuring Tremor: The Experimental Protocol

In order to assess tremor characteristics we studied its behavior in 31 patients suffering from different pathologies (Table 2.2). The average age of patients was 52.3 years old (ranging from 23 to 84 years old). All patients provided their written consent for the experiments.

Table 2.2 Description of the type of disorders and tremors investigated. The way that patients expressed the tremor is also included, for instance, patients with essential disorder expressed the tremor during voluntary muscle contraction (VMC).

Disorder	Type of tremor	Number of patients	Expression
Essential	Postural and Kinetic	21	VMC
Cerebellar	Kinetic	4	VMC
Parkinson	Parkinsonian	3	at rest
Others	Postural, kinetic and Rest	3	VMC

The diagnosis of the condition of patients was given by the neurological staff of the General Hospital of Valencia (GHV, Spain) and the functional state of patients was evaluated by means of the Faher scale, [39]. Ethical approval for this research has been granted by the Ethical Committee of the GHV.

2.4.1.1 Sensors

There is a continuous need to develop miniaturized systems with low energy consumption for biomechanical analysis that can extract a wide range of parameters from human motion. Kinematic data obtained by biomechanical studies have been increasingly used and required in active prosthetics/orthotics control systems, [111].

The tremor was detected by a customized sensor, [91, 115], which is based on the combination of two independent gyroscopes placed distally and proximally to the joint of interest. The joint angular speed is obtained by subtraction of the angular speed measured by one gyroscope from the angular speed measured by the other one. The weight of the system is roughly 15 g, [111], which is a low-mass system when compared to other sensors used in the field, for instance, [36] employed a 15 g triaxial piezoresistive accelerometer secured to a 57 g plastic splint in his experiments. The use of a low-mass sensor is important to reduce the effect of low-pass filtering on the detected signal. Further discussion about this issue is presented in [36, 111].

This system could measure the upper limb joint angle, velocity and acceleration without any external reference. Unlike accelerometers, the measurement of angular velocity is not influenced by gravity and they are in general accurate both in frequency and amplitude.

The main advantages of this system is that it is light, cheap and does not cause any discomfort to subjects thus providing a powerful tool to monitor biomechanical variables during physiological tremor movements.

2.4.1.2 Gyroscope Placement

Since gyroscope provides absolute angular velocity in its active axis, the combination of two independent gyroscopes was used. They were placed distally and proximally to the joint of interest. Gyroscopes could be placed anywhere along the same plane on the same segment providing almost identical signals. The gyroscopes could therefore be attached to a convenient position in order to avoid areas of skin and muscle movement, [91]. Figure 2.1 illustrates the placement of the gyroscopes.

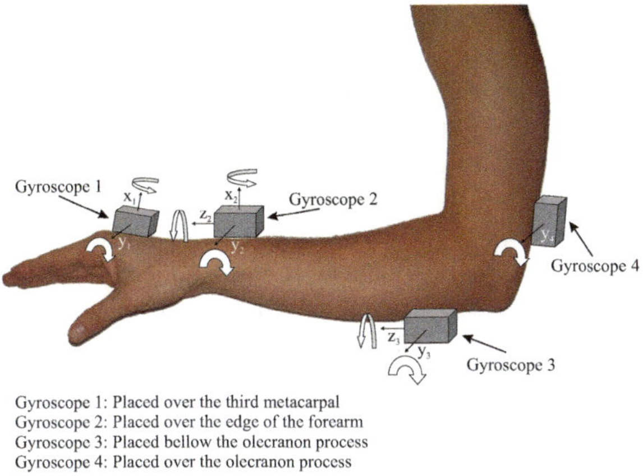

Fig. 2.1 Strategy for positioning of sensors on the upper limb of patients. The weight of the system is roughly 15g and do not influence the tremorous movement of the patient.

With gyroscopes positioned as indicated in Figure 2.1 the following movements of the upper limb were measured:

- Elbow flex-extension
- Forearm pron-supination
- Wrist flex-extension
- Wrist deviation

These articulations were selected because they are considered the most important articulations in the kinematic chain of the upper limb, [115].

2.4.1.3 Tasks

Six different tasks were employed for excitation of tremor. They are defined as follows:

1. Rest: the patient was asked to keep the arms in a rest position with the hands resting on the thighs (elbow flexed at 90° and the shoulder at 0° and hands in pronation).
2. Reaching for an object: patients had to point at a target (at the shoulder height) located in front of them. They were asked to perform the movement slowly. The distance between the shoulder and the tip of the middle finger was 85% of upper limb length.

3. Drawing a spiral: the patient was asked to follow with the index finger a spiral drawn in a sheet of paper fixed in front of them.
4. Arm outstretched: the patient was asked to maintain the upper limbs outstretched in front of them, hands in supination, against the gravity, for 30 seconds.
5. Touching nose: the patient was asked to touch the nose with the index finger, starting from a rest position (hand on the thigh). They had to keep the finger on the nose during 10 seconds.
6. Moving a cup: the patient was asked to take a rigid cup with one hand and move it to the left and to the right. They were sitting near to a white table. The target locations were identified by black tape fixed on the table. The tape was fixed along a line passing through positions defined as DEL and DER. The patient was first asked to maintain the elbow flexed at 90° and the shoulder at 0°, close to the trunk in the frontal plane. Hands were in pronation on the table with fingers extended. The targets were located at 10 cm on the left and on the right from the extremity of the third finger (DE left and DE right). Areas of the position of the cup were pre-drawn with a red marker.

In all tasks the patient was sitting on a chair. This set of tasks aims to activate all different types of tremor. Figure 2.2 illustrates a patient performing the six tasks presented above.

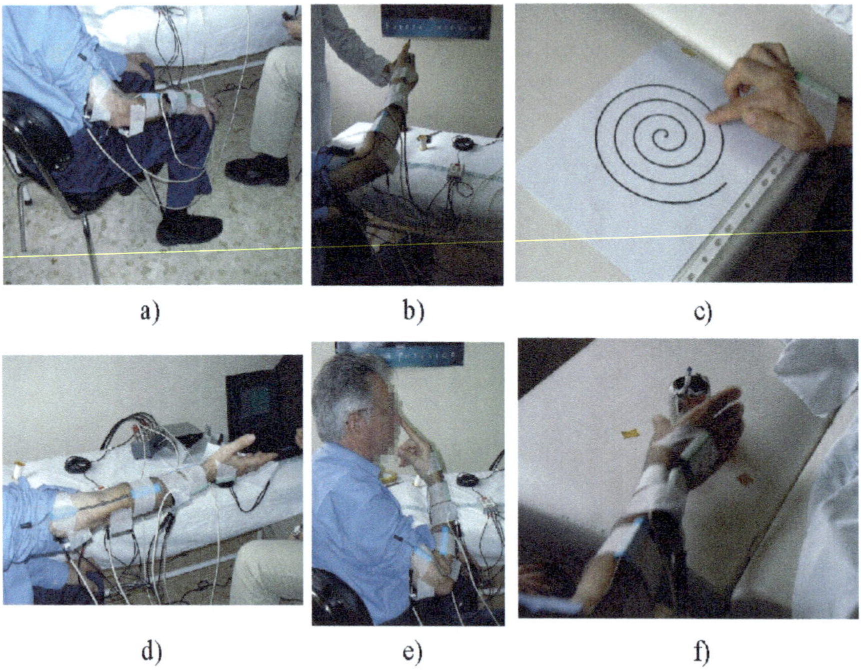

Fig. 2.2 Tasks of the measurement session: a) Rest, b) Reaching for an object, c) Drawing spiral, d) Arm outstretched, e) Touching nose, f) Moving a cup.

2.4.2 *Studying Tremor: The Hilbert Spectrum*

The generation of the Hilbert Spectrum (HS) is performed into two steps. First, the Empirical Mode Decomposition (EMD) decomposes the input time-series into a set of functions designated as Intrinsic Mode Function (IMFs), and secondly those functions are used for generation of a 3-D plot called the Hilbert Spectrum. The following sections provide a description of the constituent steps of the HA.

2.4.2.1 The Empirical Mode Decomposition

The main aim of the EMD is to decompose a time-series into a set of components or functions, known as IMFs. This class of function was defined in [61]. To be considered an IMF a time-series has to satisfy two conditions: first, in the whole data set, the number of extrema and the number of zero crossings must be either equal or differ at most by one, and secondly, at any point, the mean value of the envelope defined by the local maxima and the envelope defined by the local minima is zero.

Note that the decomposition of a time-series into IMFs consists in the identification of the basic units (IMFs) in that time-series. A practical procedure, known as sifting process, is employed for this purpose, [61]. It involves the following steps, leading to a decomposition of the signal S(t) into its constituent IMFs:

a) x (an auxiliary variable) is set to the signal to be analyzed and a variable k, which is the number of estimated IMFs, is set to zero.

b) Splines are fitted to the upper extrema and the lower extrema. This will define the lower (LE) and upper envelopes (UE).

c) The average envelope, m, is calculated as the arithmetic mean between UE and LE.

d) A candidate IMF, h, is estimated as the difference between x and m.

e) If h does not fulfill the criteria defining an IMF, it is assigned to the variable x and the steps *b*) to *d*) are repeated. Otherwise, if h is an IMF then the procedure moves to step *f*).

f) If h is an IMF it is saved as c_k, where k is the k*th* component.

g) The mean squared error, *mse*, between two consecutive IMFs c_{k-1} and c_k, is calculated, and this value is compared to a stopping condition (usually a very small value, i.e. 10^{-5}).

h) If the stopping condition is not reached, the partial residue, r_k, is estimated as the difference between a previous partial residue r_{k-1} and c_k, and its content is assigned to the dummy variable x and the steps of **b**) to **d**) are repeated.

i) If the stopping condition is reached then the sifting process is finalized and the final residue r_{final} can be estimated as the difference between $S(t)$ and the sum of all IMFs.

Note that the criterion used to state whether h is an IMF or not is to verify if h satisfies the two conditions that define an IMF.

An important feature of the sifting process is that it, adaptively and based solely on the data, is able to find appropriate time-scales that may reveal important information embedded in the original signal. In fact, single IMFs may have a physical meaning, and an important issue in any practical application is to determine the existence of this meaning.

2.4.2.2 Hibert Spectrum Generation

Once IMFs are obtained as result of the sifting process, it is possible to generate the Hilbert Spectrum, or a 3-D plot (time-frequency-energy) that represents the variation of frequency and energy of IMFs over time. The notion of frequency and energy for each IMF is obtained by employing the concept of analytic signals.

An analytic signal is a complex signal with one-sided spectrum that preserves all information contained in the original signal, [86]. Note that the representation of a real signal as an analytical signal eliminates redundancy, since the negative half of the signal frequency spectrum containing redundant information with respect to the positive half is eliminated. A very simple way of estimating an analytical signal is by employing the Hilbert Transform, [86]. The real part of an analytical signal is the original input time-series, whereas its complex component is the Hilbert Transform of that signal.

Given an analytic signal, $Z(t)$, defined as $Z(t) = X(t) + iY(t) = a(t)e^{j\theta(t)}$, where $X(t)$ is the input time-series and $Y(t)$ the Hilbert Transform of $X(t)$, the following instantaneous attributes of $Z(t)$ can be defined:

$$a(t) = [X(t)^2 + Y(t)^2]^{1/2} \tag{2.4}$$

$$\theta(t) = \arctan\left(\frac{Y(t)}{X(t)}\right) \tag{2.5}$$

$$\omega(t) = \frac{d\theta(t)}{dt} \tag{2.6}$$

where $a(t)$ is the instantaneous amplitude, $\theta(t)$ is the instantaneous phase and $\omega(t)$ is the instantaneous frequency.

With the definition of instantaneous attributes above the Hilbert Spectrum, $H(\omega,t)$, is generated as follows:

1. Estimate intrinsic mode functions from the input signal.
2. Estimate the instantaneous attributes of each IMF.
3. Generate a 3-D plot, $H(\omega,t)$, in which the amplitude is contoured in the time-frequency plane.

In contrast to other time-frequency methods, the HS does not define an explicit equation that maps a 1-D time-series into a 3-D representation that provides information about time, frequency and energy (amplitude).

From the HS it is also possible to estimate the Marginal Hilbert Spectrum (MHS), $h(\omega)$, which is defined in Equation 2.7. In practice $h(\omega)$ is analogous to the Fourier power spectrum.

$$h(\omega) = \int_0^T H(\omega,t)dt \tag{2.7}$$

2.4.2.3 Data Analysis

Figure 2.3 depicts the sequence of steps for data analysis. The resulting movement profile (or the collected signal x) was sampled at 400 Hz and filtered using a 5th order low-pass FIR filter with cut off frequency set to 20 Hz. This is relevant for attenuation of the influence of any high-frequency noise on the digitized signal y.

In a further step, y was manually decomposed into tremor and voluntary activity, by means of a digital pass-band Butterworth filter. Note that the word manually (or manual) refers to the ad hoc setting of the the cutoff frequencies of the digital filter in contrast to an automatic setting provided by adaptive methods like the EMD.

For estimation of the voluntary movement, VM_{ref}, the cutoff frequencies of this filter was set to 0 - 2 Hz. The cutoff frequencies employed for detection of the tremor, T_{ref}, were 2 - 20 Hz. Previous investigation of this data set showed that the tremor activity was limited between 3 Hz and 8 Hz, [108], and that voluntary movements were always below 2 Hz for the tasks described above. It is well established in the literature of tremor that the voluntary movement and tremor movement used

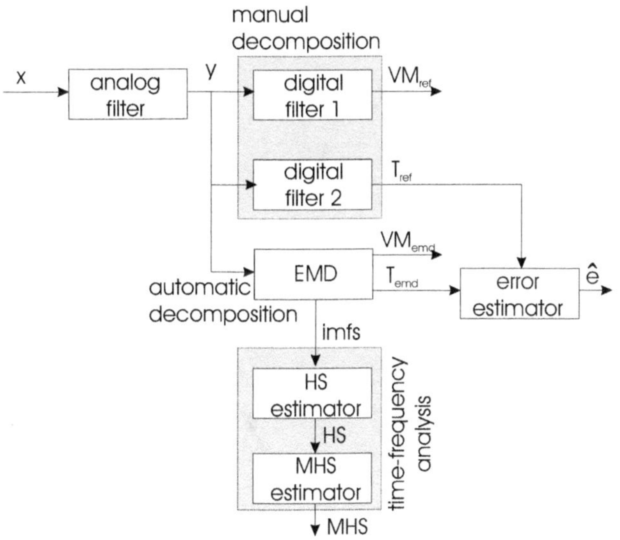

Fig. 2.3 Block diagram showing the sequence of analyses performed in this study. First the detected signal x was filtered and digitized in order to yield the time-series y. In a further step this signal was decomposed into tremor (T_{ref}) and voluntary movement (VM_{ref}). This was manually performed by means of two distinct digital filters. The same signal y was also automatically decomposed via EMD, and the automatically estimated tremor T_{emd} was compared to T_{ref}. The components provided by the EMD, or $imfs$, were employed for a further analysis of the signal y in the frequency domain.

to be separated in frequency. Tremor (2-12 Hz) tends to be at higher frequencies than voluntary (0-2 Hz) movements, [33, 107]. Note that those digital filters do not introduce phase lag in the filtered signal.

The time-series y was also automatically decomposed via EMD. This decomposition yielded intrinsic mode functions from which it was possible to identify the tremor T_{emd} and voluntary movement VM_{emd}. A comparison between T_{emd} and T_{ref} was performed and resulted in the generation of the estimated square error signal $\hat{e} = \sqrt{(T_{ref} - T_{emd})^2}$. This signal measured the discrepancy between automatic and manual estimates. A small value for $\hat{e}$ indicates a strong relation between an intrinsic mode function (T_{emd}) and a manual definition of tremor (T_{ref}). Thus, in practice, a small $\hat{e}$ is a good evidence that T_{emd} has a physical meaning related to tremor activity. The identification of such a physical meaning is the main focus of this study.

An additional investigation showing how the activities of tremor and voluntary movement were perceived in the frequency domain was also performed. For this purpose, the HS and MHS were employed as indicated in Figure 2.3.

Figure 2.4 shows an example of a signal manually decomposed into its constituents, i.e. the voluntary movement and tremor.

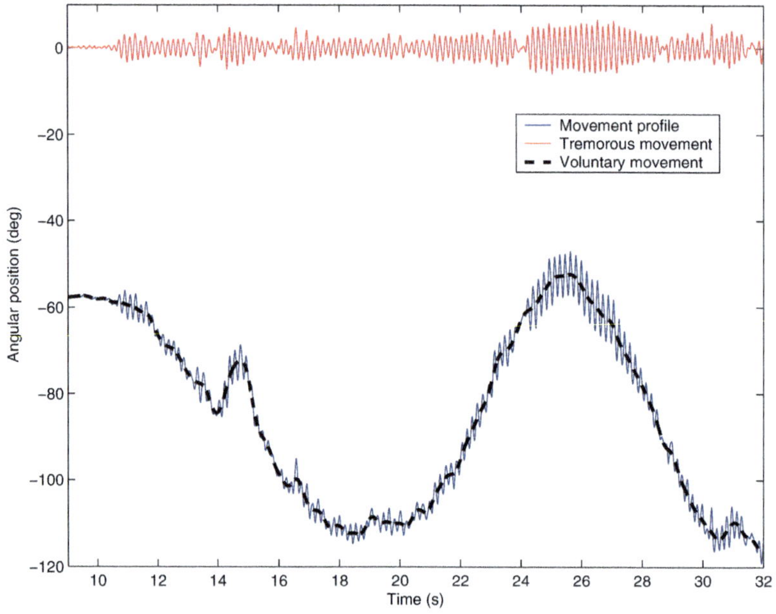

Fig. 2.4 Example of manual decomposition of the movement profile (x) of an Essential tremor patient performing the task of drawing a spiral. Digital filters are employed for estimation of tremulous movement (T_{ref}), oscillating around zero in the top, and voluntary movement (VM_{ref}).

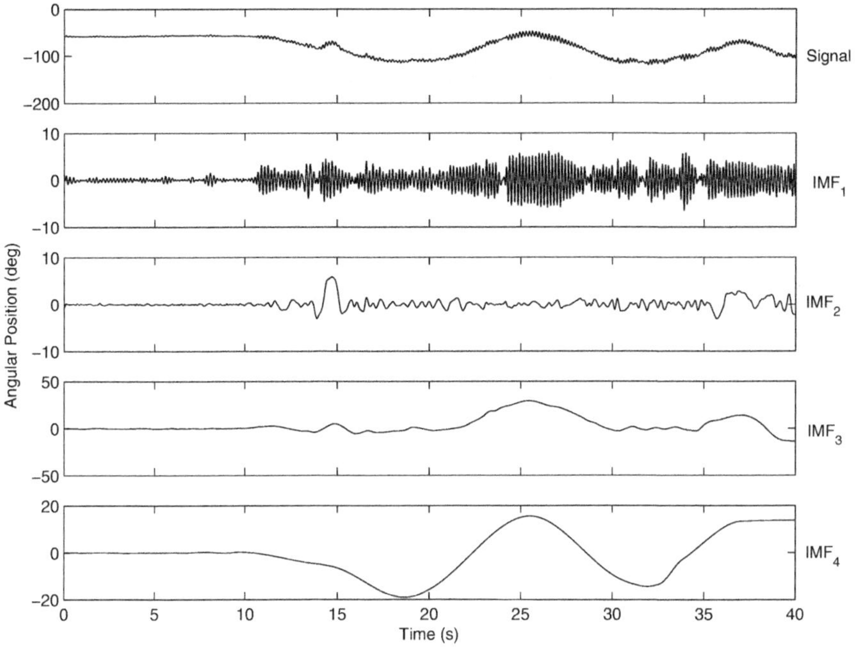

Fig. 2.5 Decomposition of a movement profile (Signal) detected from an Essential tremor patient provided by EMD. Four intrinsic mode function ($IMF_1,\ldots,IMF_4$) were obtained. IMF_1 was identified as the tremulous movement.

2.4.2.4 Automatic Detection of Tremor

The signal presented in Figure 2.5 (top) was detected from a patient with Essential tremor performing the draw spiral test. The signal components, or intrinsic mode functions, obtained by means of the EMD are also shown in this figure. The first component identified as IMF_1 is the finest time-scale component, whereas the last component (IMF_4) is the largest time-scale component.

A comparative study between different IMFs and the tremor signal (obtained manually) showed that the IMF_1, which is the component that best represents the high frequencies of the signal, was an accurate estimate of the tremor, i.e. this component had a very strong physical meaning. This observation is illustrated in Figure 2.6. The manual estimate of the tremor is in the top of the figure, its automatic estimate, or IMF_1, is in the middle, and the estimated error, $\hat{e}$, between those two signals is shown in the bottom. Note that the error is very small.

The same analysis for the signal in Figure 2.5 was carried out for all available data sets. It was also noted that the voluntary movement can be obtained by the summation of all available IMFs but the first one, which represented the tremor (see Figure 2.7).

This investigation showed that the first IMF was always a precise estimate of the tremor. This accuracy was quantified by the mean square error signal, $\bar{e} = mean(\hat{e})$.

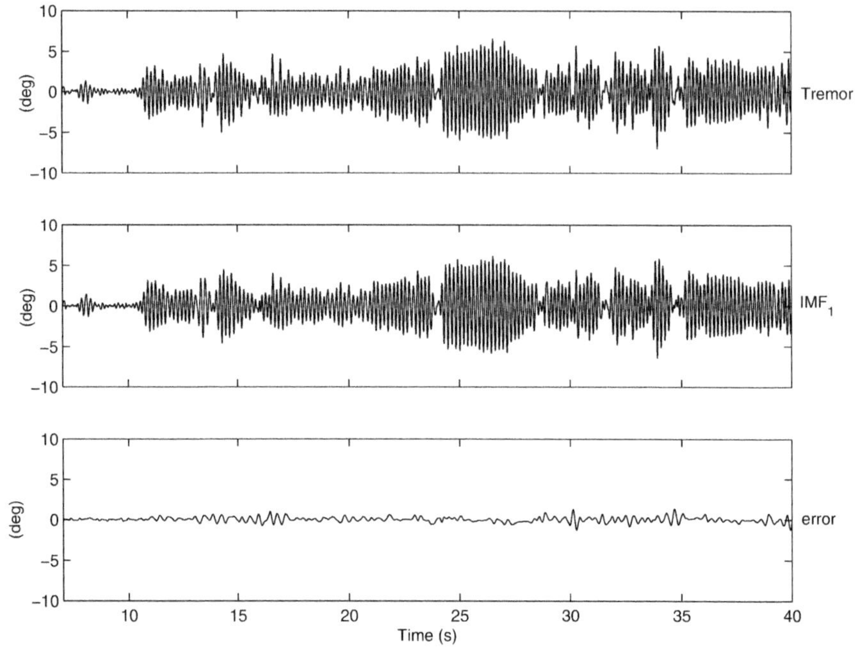

Fig. 2.6 Comparison between IMF_1 (from Figure 2.5) and the manual estimate of the tremor (T_{ref}). Note that the error signal is very small.

The average and standard deviation of distinct signal errors $\bar{e}$ was estimated. The results show that a very small error, 0.09 ± 0.19 degrees, was obtained for all pathologies. Note that due to fact the majority of patients suffers from Essential tremor the results are only statistically significant for the tremor activity related to this pathology. Nevertheless, the results indicates that the method is able to estimate tremor activity for all pathologies evaluated. Additional investigation should be pursued in order to validate the performance of this technique in the estimation of tremorous movements from others pathologies.

2.4.2.5 Visualization of Tremor on the Hilbert Spectrum

It has been shown that a particular intrinsic function is physically related to the tremor. Besides the representation of embedded components in the signal those functions may also be employed for a time-frequency analysis of time-series. This is obtained via the Hilbert Spectrum.

In practice it was observed that the Hilbert Spectrum could describe the variation of the energy and frequency of tremor and voluntary movement activities distinctly. That is, the energy of tremor and voluntary movement was very well localized in time and frequency. This is illustrated in Figures 2.8 and 2.9 for patients with different disorders. The oscillations around 5 Hz are related to tremor activities whereas the others are related to other components of the global movement.

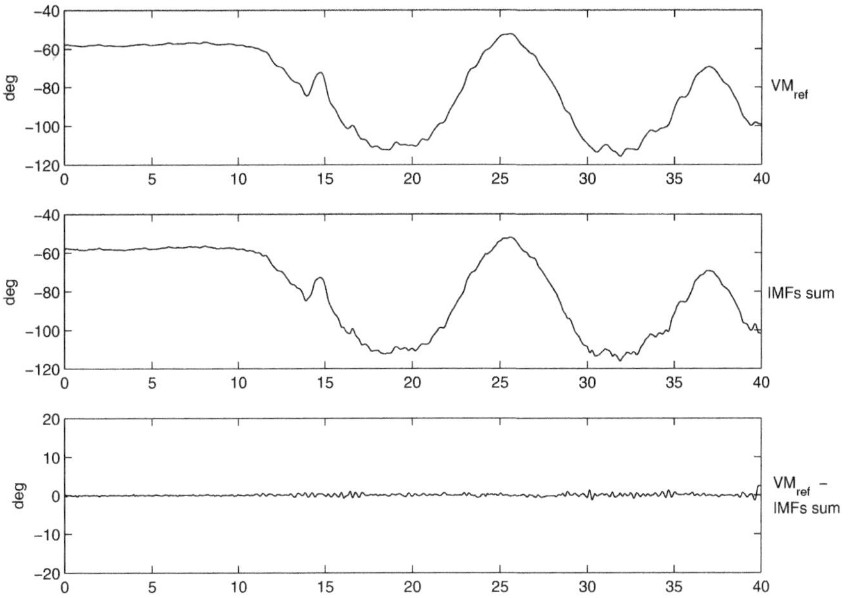

Fig. 2.7 Comparison between voluntary motion (top) and its estimate obtained via summation of different IMFs (IMF_2, IMF_3, IMF_4) (middle) shown in Figure 2.5. Note that the difference between the manual and the automatic estimation of the voluntary movement $(V_{ref} - IMFs$ sum) is very small (bottom).

In these figures the Spectrogram was also included for comparison with the HS. From their analysis it is possible to conclude that the Spectrogram allows for a global description of the energy of the signal, whereas the HS provides information about local changes of energy over time.

2.4.2.6 Analysis of the Power Based on the MHS

The integration of the HS over the time results in the MHS. The MHS describes how the signal energy varies as function of the frequency. Figure 2.10 shows the MHS for a patient with essential tremor performing the task of touching the nose. Note that the distribution provided by the MHS is bimodal and that its first peak is related to the voluntary movement, whereas the second is the energy of tremor activity.

2.4.2.7 Discussion

In this section, an analysis of the results of the above proposed methodology is reported. We mainly focus on the application of Empirical Mode Decomposition as a new tool for the study of tremor time series. EMD has been identified as a very useful tool for an automatic decomposition of the signal into tremor and voluntary signal.

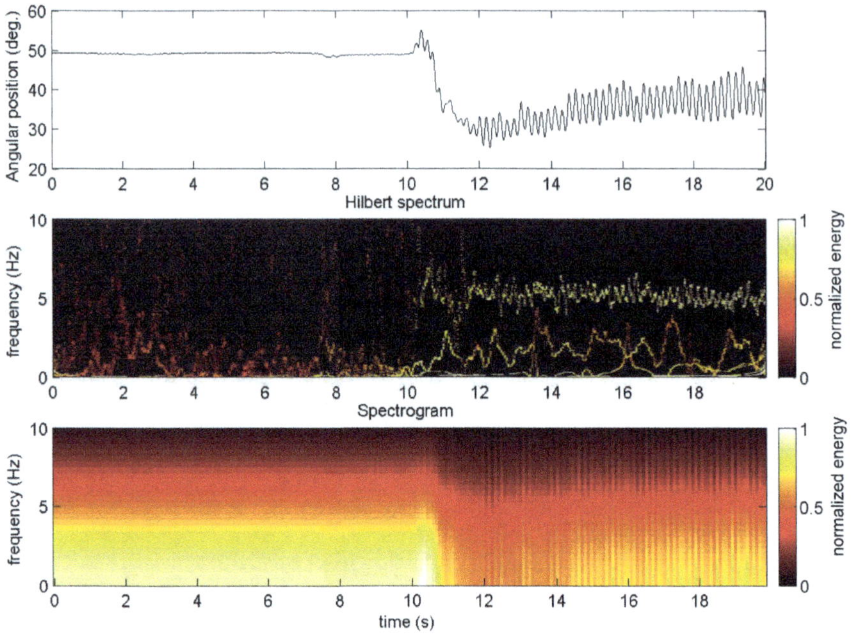

Fig. 2.8 Hilbert Spectrum and Spectrogram of an Essential tremor patient performing the task of keeping the arms outstretched. Note that the energy of the involuntary movement is clearly separated from the energy of the voluntary movement on the HS. This separation is not so evident on the Spectrogram. The high levels of energy activity on the HS could be perceived when the patient is performing the task.

The results presented showed that the first IMF could accurately estimate the tremor. This was observed in the whole data set, which had more than 2000 samples of signals with tremor activity, collected from 31 patients performing 6 different tasks.

Currently, there is no available technique that can accurately model the tremor, [108, 129]. Most of methodologies are based on the assumption that the tremor is stationary or is similar to sine wave. The fact that the tremor time series could be described by an intrinsic mode function states that the tremor signal, for all patients considered in this study, satisfies two conditions, [61]: 1) in the whole data set, the number of extrema and the number of zero crossings must be either equal or differ at most by one; 2) At any point, the mean value of the envelope defined by the local maxima and the envelope defined by the local minima is zero. These observations suggest that any investigation concerning the modelling of tremor should take into account those properties.

The major discrepancies between the signal estimated by EMD (IMF_1) and the tremor manually decomposed (T_{ref}) were found in the patients with no diagnosed tremor. This may be explained by the fact that in those patients the movement profile was also corrupted by other involuntary movements besides tremor, such as spasms. Spasms are a non-tremorous type of involuntary movement aperiodic, erratic, unpredictable at our current state of understanding, and can overlap in frequency with

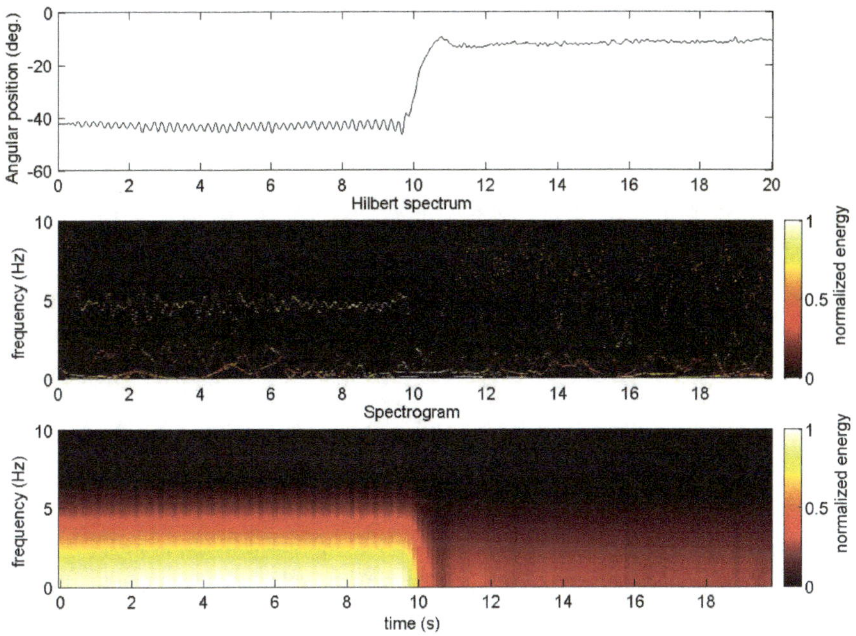

Fig. 2.9 Hilbert Spectrum and Spectrogram of a Parkinson tremor patient performing the task of reaching for an object. The Spectrogram could not show local variation of energy. Note that different from the HS presented in Figure 2.8 the energy of the tremor is concentrated when the limbs are at rest, or within the first 10 s. This is a characteristic of Parkinsonian patients.

voluntary motion. These movements can occur at higher frequencies overlapping the tremor frequency. In addition, these involuntary movements present an unstable and non-stationary behavior. This highlights the fact that in practice, any manual or arbitrary decomposition based on pre-fixed band-pass filters, might result in a inaccurate estimate of the tremor movement or any other relevant physiological event (e.g. spasms), see Figure 2.5.

A more detailed analysis of the IMF components indicates that the second IMF could estimate non-tremorous type of involuntary movements, such as spasms or pathological myoclonus [108], see Figure 2.5 where the spasm movement present at time $t = 15$ s is highlighted in the IMF_2. The automatic identification of these movements is very important in order to help their understanding, as to date there is no technique able to identify these movements. Further investigation correlating the signal provided by EMD estimation of spasmodic movements and EMG signals from the muscles that execute these movements will be carried out in order to validate this supposition.

Having obtained the intrinsic mode function components, the Hilbert transform can be applied to each component and the instantaneous frequency can be computed, according to equations (1), (2) and (3). The Hilbert Spectrum enables the representation of the amplitude and the instantaneous frequency of the input signal as function

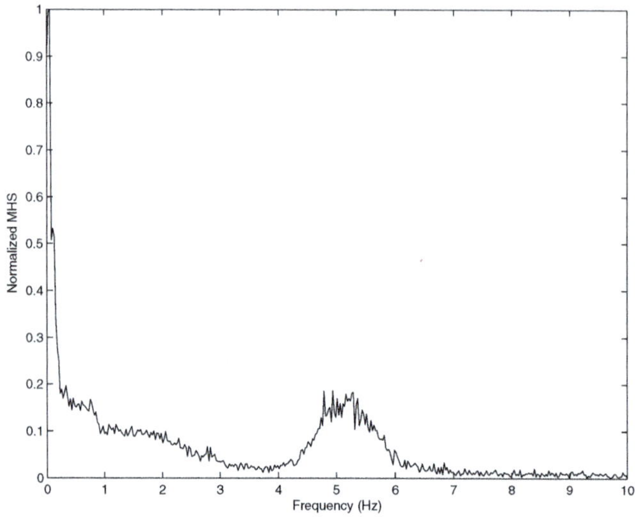

Fig. 2.10 Marginal Hilbert Spectrum estimated from the signal shown in Figure 2.8. This energy is bimodal indicating the clear separation between voluntary and tremor in frequency domain.

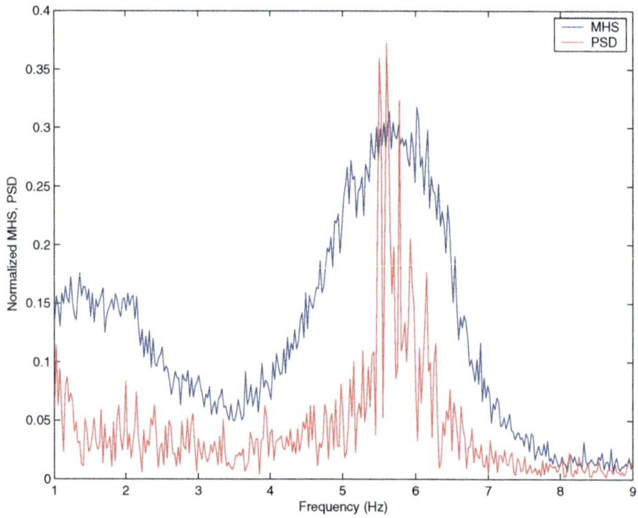

Fig. 2.11 Comparison between power spectrum based on the Fourier Transform with the Marginal Hilbert Spectrum (MHS), estimated from the signal in Figure 2.8 detected from an Essential tremor patient performing the task of keeping the arms outstretched.

of time in which the amplitude could be contoured on the time-frequency plane. Since the tremorous movements is well described by the first IMF, this method is a very useful tool for visualization of energy activity of tremor.

The description of the energy of the tremor on the HS is important because it allows for a good visualization of how the frequency and energy of the tremor vary over time. With this tool it is possible to clearly identify the onset and offset of tremor activity, as well as its frequency and amplitude changes over the time, see Figures 2.8 and 2.9. These techniques could be very useful to perform objective measurements of any kind of tremor and can therefore be used to perform tremor functional assessment.

Due to its oscillatory characteristic, tremor is well suited to spectral analysis such as the Fourier Transform, which is the most popular method of tremor quantification, [37, 108]. FFT-based spectral methods model the input signal as stationary periodic signal. Yet tremor amplitude and frequency are time-varying, [33, 34, 107, 108], and therefore it is desirable to develop quantitative methods which do not assume stationarity. The Marginal Hilbert Spectrum offers a measure of the total amplitude (or energy) contribution from each frequency value over the entire data span being able to precisely detect the energy activities of tremor and voluntary movements. In the Fourier representation, the existence of energy at a frequency, ω, means a component of a sine or a cosine wave persisted through the time span of the data. Here, the existence of energy at a frequency, ω, means only that, in the whole time span of data, there is a greater likelihood for such wave to have appeared locally. Figure 2.11 shows a comparison between the Fourier Spectrum and the marginal Hilbert Spectrum. It is clear that the MHS give us a more precise spectrum, i.e. without energy spreading.

2.4.3 Tremor Study Based on Empirical Mode Decomposition

Based on this technique, a study of the tremorous movement at different joints of the upper limb was developed. The study was performed with the data collect from the experiments introduced in the previous section and aim at understanding tremorous behaviour. The main conclusions of this study are the following:

1. The amplitude of the tremorous movement is larger in distal joints than in proximal joints. For instance, tremor at elbow joints are smaller than at wrist joints.
2. The frequency of tremorous movements is comprised in the bandwidth between 3 and 8 Hz.
3. Tremor frequency at different joints of the upper limb has very similar values.
4. Tremor frequency is not related to the task performed by the patient.
5. The frequency of tremorous movement is constant during the execution of a task, nevertheless it could change during repetitions of the same task.
6. Tremor activity is not always present during the experiments. Patients showed tremor activity just during 40% of the time measured. This highlight the importance of detecting tremor onset for its suppression.
7. Sex and age does not influence tremor behaviour.

The results of this analysis generate some very useful information about tremorous movement. The main novelty of this study is that it is centered in tremor at joint level while the majority of the studies presented in the literature are centered in the study of tremor at finger tip. Furthermore, the technique introduced allows a clear visualization of tremor activity along the time. The main drawback of this technique is the impossibility to implement it in real-time. In order to address this issue, next chapter describes the development of an algorithm able to distinguish in real-time tremorous movement from voluntary movement.

2.4.4 Study of Tremor Characteristics Based on a Biomechanical Model of the Upper Limb

This section introduces an estimation of tremor kinematic parameters, reproducing upper limb kinematics based on a biomechanical model. The method used for analysis of tremorous movements is based on a combination of solid modelling techniques with anthropometric models of the upper limb, from which a kinematic and dynamic upper limb model can be developed. This model of upper limb musculoskeletal systems can be used to estimate the force contribution of each muscle component during motion, to experiment with modifications of musculoskeletal topology and to devise complex motion coordination strategies. The input to the model is the angular position, velocity and acceleration of each joint, measured by gyroscopes placed on the upper limbs of patients suffering from tremor.

The input of this model was the data obtained from the patients introduced in section 2.4.1.

2.4.4.1 Biomechanical Model of the Upper-Arm

A biomechanical model of the upper arm was built taking into account the Leva and Zatsiorsky and Seluyanov tables, [75], in order to describe its kinematics and dynamics. These tables are one of the most widely accepted means of performing dynamic analysis in the field of biomechanics, in particular in sports and medical biomechanics. Leva adjustments were made in order to accurately define the anthropometric measurements required to obtain inertial parameters from Zatsiorsky tables.

A solid rigid model of the forearm was built with the information from the above mentioned tables and parameterized following the Denavit-Hartenberg approach. In addition, a library was created to permit dynamic analysis of the system. This analysis was performed using the recursive algorithm, [42], so that the libraries could be built on a modular basis.

2.4.4.2 Denavit–Hartenberg Parametrization

The model proposed considers the upper limb as a chain composed of three rigid bodies – the arm, the forearm and the hand – articulated on the rigid base formed by the trunk and linked by ideal rotational joints, [88]. This representation relies on three assumptions: 1) the mechanical behaviour of the upper limb with respect to the trunk is independent of the rest of the human body; 2) each segment, including bones and soft tissues, has similar rigid body motions; and 3) the deformation of the soft tissues does not significantly affect the mechanical properties of a segment as a whole.

The hand was considered as a rigid extension of the forearm on the assumption that hand motion has a negligible effect on the broad motion dynamics of the upper limb. This made it necessary to determine a rigid body equivalent to the hand and forearm assembly to be substituted in the rigid body dynamic analysis. As a result, four rigid segments were defined in order to be able to analyse all the recorded degrees of freedom. Each segment is responsible for a degree of freedom: 1) elbow flexion-extension; 2) pronation-supination; 3) wrist flexion-extension; 4) wrist deviation.

Two of these segments are virtual (no mass and no length). Each segment has its own reference system (plus a coordinate frame for the all of them) attached. Figure 2.12 shows the coordinate frames defined and the degree of freedom represented for each system.

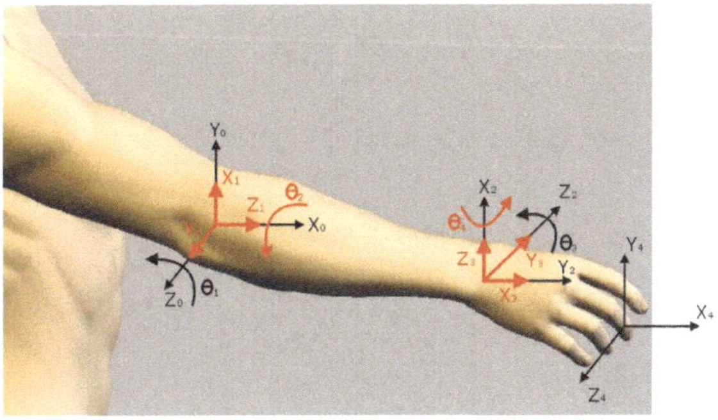

Fig. 2.12 Solid model representation of the forearm.

The Denavit-Hartenberg parameters can be seen in table 2.3. For rotary elements, the parameter θ determines the position of the joint. The table then indicates the relationship between the parameter and the physiological measured angle represented by β_i for each segment i. F_L means forearm length and H_L means hand length.

Table 2.3 DH parameters.

Segment	d	a	θ	α
1 - Elbow F/E	0	0	$\beta_1+\pi/2$	$\pi/2$
2 - Pronation	F_L	0	β_2	$\pi/2$
3 - Wrist F/E	0	0	$\beta_3+\pi/2$	$\pi/2$
4 - Elbow Dev.	0	H_L	β_4	$\pi/2$

2.4.4.3 Biomechanical Parameters per Segment

Biomechanical parameters per segment were obtained from [75]. Segment 1 and Segment 3 are virtual; they are only defined to cope with the degrees of freedom of elbow flexion-extension and wrist flexion-extension respectively. However, when these segments are moved, the masses of the "real" segments are moved. All the inertial and mass parameters of a segment are defined below, using the following symbols: B_M, body mass, F_L, forearm length, F_M, forearm mass, H_L, hand length, H_M, hand mass, CoG_M, centre of gravity of each segment (obtained from Leva tables), and MI inertia matrix.

$$\begin{aligned}
M_1 &= 0\\
CoG_1 &= [0,0,0]\\
MI_1 &= \begin{bmatrix} 0\,0\,0\\ 0\,0\,0\\ 0\,0\,0 \end{bmatrix}\\
M_2 &= F_M = 1.6 \cdot \frac{B_M}{100}\\
CoG_2 &= [0, F_L(0.457-1), 0]\\
MI_2 &= \begin{bmatrix} 0.08 & 0 & 0\\ 0 & 0.09 & 0\\ 0 & 0 & 0.15 \end{bmatrix} \cdot F_M \cdot F_L^2
\end{aligned} \tag{2.8}$$

$$\begin{aligned}
M_3 &= 0\\
CoG_3 &= [0,0,0]\\
MI_3 &= \begin{bmatrix} 0\,0\,0\\ 0\,0\,0\\ 0\,0\,0 \end{bmatrix}\\
M_4 &= = M_M = 0.6 \cdot \frac{B_M}{100}\\
CoG_4 &= [0, H_L(0.79-1), 0]\\
MI_4 &= \begin{bmatrix} 0.55 & 0 & 0\\ 0 & 0.42 & 0\\ 0 & 0 & 0.66 \end{bmatrix} \cdot H_M \cdot H_L^2
\end{aligned} \tag{2.9}$$

The computational algorithm used is based on the Newton-Euler equations of motion described in [42]. Thanks to their recursive implementation, these equations of motion are the most efficient set of computational equations for running on a uniprocessor computer, so that implementation in real-time is possible.

2.4.4.4 Results

This analysis is intended to estimate the torque and power of the tremorous movement in each joint of the upper limb based on the information provided by the gyroscopes.

Active orthoses are intended to counteract tremor by applying controlled forces. Torque is an essential parameter in the choice of the actuator technology that will be used by powered orthoses. Special care should be taken with this parameter since it presents a dynamic behaviour. As can be seen in Figure 2.13, this parameter presents a dynamic behavior. The actuator technology that will drive the orthosis must be able to apply the same torque characteristics. Table 2.4 summarizes the mean value of torque estimated in each joint of the upper limb for the tasks of stretching out the arm and putting finger to nose. These tasks are shown because they are the ones in which maximum values of tremor activity were registered.

The other important parameter is the power that the device can absorb. The amount of power consumed in relation to tremor is one of the key parameters that need to be taken into account in the design of these devices. The power at the joint plus the performance of the devices will also determine the battery capacity. Tremor

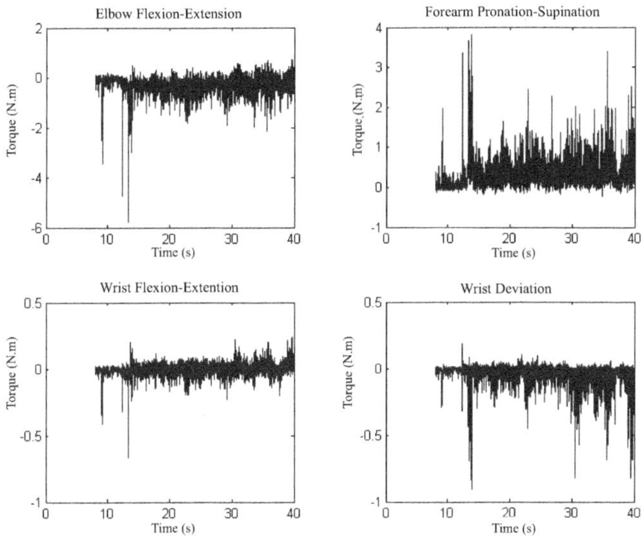

Fig. 2.13 Arm outstretched torques.

Table 2.4 Mean values of the torque estimated in finger to nose and outstretched arm tasks.

Movement	Finger to nose	Outstretched Arm
Elbow Flexo-extension	1.9 $N.m$	1.2 $N.m$
Forearm Prono-supination	3.7 $N.m$	1.9 $N.m$
Wrist Flexo-extension	0.4 $N.m$	0.2 $N.m$
Wrist Deviation	1.1 $N.m$	0.5 $N.m$

is assumed to be a stationary movement and, leaving aside the viscous coefficient of joint braking, there is no effective work done on the joint. That is why the RMS value of the power estimated for the tremorous movement during the putting finger to nose and stretching out arm tasks are presented in Table 2.5.

Table 2.5 RMS values of the power estimated in each joint during execution of finger to nose and outstretched arm tasks.

Movement	Finger to nose	Outstretched arm
Elbow Flexo-extension	0.2W	0.01W
Forearm Prono-supination	1.8W	0.2W
Wrist Flexo-extension	0.08W	0.03W
Wrist Deviation	0.4W	0.04W

The results of this study show the basis of the dynamics of tremorous movement in each joint of the upper limb, information that is required for the design of portable active upper limb exoskeletons.

2.5 Conclusions

This chapter introduced a detailed review of tremor thorough literature review in the topic of technological management of pathologic tremor, specifically focused on upper extremity tremor. Tremor is still an unknown issue. Physiological tremor has been studied in detail, and is quite well described in the literature, but there are still some mismatches between different authors about its origins. The pathological kinds of tremor are less known than physiological tremor. Some kinds of pathological tremors are better described (i.e. Parkinson tremor), but again aetiology is unknown in most cases.

There is no consensus in the optimal way to objectively measure tremor in the upper limb. In this chapter the authors proposed a new approach for tremor assessment based on gyroscopes. Morevoer, a novel tool for the analysis of tremor time series is introduced. The main advantage of this technique it that it allows an automatic estimate of the tremorous movement in the different pathologies considered in this study. Additional investigation should be pursued in order to validate the performance of this technique in the estimation of tremorous movements from others pathologies.

The technique presented is a high-resolution method that overcomes some of the limitations of Fourier based analysis, which is the standard technique to the study of tremor time series. However, a detailed comparative study considering the HS and other joint time-frequency distributions (e.g. Spectrogram, Scalogram, Autoregressive models, Wigner-Ville distribution) should be performed, in the study of tremor, to better understand the advantages and disadvantages of these techniques. Independent of such a study this research has shown that the HS has a promising application in the analysis of tremor.

The application of this technique introduces new attributes to the tremorous signal such as instantaneous amplitude, instantaneous phase and instantaneous frequency. This attributes opens the research field in the tremor field. Future work will be focused on the use of these parameters as parameters for the diagnosis of tremor pathologies.

Based on this new methodology, a study of tremor behaviour at joint level was performed and is presented in this chapter. This study brings new knowledge to the tremor field and pave the way for the development of upper limb exoskeletons for tremor suppression.

Chapter 3
Upper Limb Exoskeleton for Tremor Suppression: Cognitive HR Interaction

This book describes a new method for tremor suppression by means of a wearable exoskeleton that estimates in realtime the amount of biomechanical load to be applied. Therefore, it is in this field of rehabilitation robotics for tremor suppression that estimation of instantaneous tremor amplitude and frequency becomes mandatory, as it is necessary to obtain reliable tremor models that generate effective suppression commands. In addition to being important to distinguish between desired and undesired motion, the analysis of the tremor signal, both in terms of frequency and amplitude, is relevant to assess the stationary characteristics of tremor, i.e. frequency drift and amplitude variation.

To achieve satisfactory tremor suppression, the wearable robot must leave concomitant voluntary movement unmodified, compensating for tremor. The capacity of the control strategies of the exoskeleton to apply biomechanical loading on tremor while allowing the user to perform his/her voluntary movements is the core of the cognitive interaction between the exoskeleton and the human.

Regarding its aetiology, tremors are caused by the different combinations of four different mechanisms: (1) mechanically induced oscillations, (2) oscillations due to reflexes, (3) oscillations due to central neuronal circuits, and (4) oscillations because of disturbed feedback or feedforward loops, [108]. However, understanding of the origins of tremors is far from complete. Estimation of tremor parameters is fundamental for the development of more objective diagnostic tools and clinical scales, as it will enhance the objectivity, reliability, comparability and standardization of the existing ones. In fact, tremor frequency is, together with how tremor is activated and medical and family history, one of the key features for clinical classification of tremors, as agreed by the Movement Disorder Society, [29].

This chapter will introduce a new approach to estimate instantaneous tremor frequency and amplitude based on Inertial Measurement Unit (IMU) information. It consists in a two-stage algorithm that separates tremorous and voluntary motion based on their different frequency content. The two-stage algorithm consists of a voluntary motion estimation and a tremor modelling algorithm that extracts its characteristics. For both of them, different candidate algorithms are evaluated and selected according to adequate figures of merit.

E. Rocon and J.L. Pons: Exoskeletons in Rehabilitation Robotics, STAR 69, pp. 53–65.
springerlink.com

3.1 Tremor Isolation

Neurological investigations demonstrate that people with tremor undergo a change in the way they perform their volitional tasks. From a signal processing point of view, tremor may be isolated from voluntary motion based solely on frequency information, assuming that it affects volitional motion in an additive manner, [105]. Previous works report that most of the activities of daily living are carried out in a lower frequency band than tremor. For example, a large study with young and elderly healthy people and patients suffering from tremor, demonstrated that both groups were able to perform tracking tasks with a frequency up to 2 Hz, the bandwidth decreasing with age, [106]. Also, in [80] it is shown that most of the activities of daily living involve a frequency range between 0 and 1 Hz. Voluntary motion and tremor frequency bands are clearly distinguished: Voluntary movement corresponds to the frequency band below 2 Hz (most of the energy between 0 and 1 Hz) whereas tremor is centered around 5.5 Hz. It is thus possible to utilize zero phase recursive filtering techniques to isolate tremorous and voluntary motion from the recorded signal, as the EMD technique introduced in the previous chapter of this book. These techniques, however, are not real-time implementable.

A number of estimation algorithms have been developed for tremor suppression. The most used are robust algorithms based on IEEE-STD-1057, which is a standard for fitting sine waves to noisy discrete-time observations. In particular, the weighted-frequency Fourier linear combiner (WFLC) developed by Riviere, [107], in the context of actively counteracting physiological tremor in microsurgery was implemented. The WFLC is an adaptive algorithm that estimates tremor using a sinusoidal model, estimating its time-varying frequency, amplitude, and phase. The WFLC can be described by equation 3.1. It assumes that the tremor can be mathematically modelled as a pure sinusoidal signal of frequency ω_0 plus M harmonics and computes the error, ε_k, between the motion, s_k, and its harmonic model.

$$\varepsilon_k = s_k - \sum_{r=1}^{M} \left[w_{r_k} \sin(r\omega_{0_k} k) + w_{r+M_k} \cos(r\omega_{0_k} k) \right] \tag{3.1}$$

In its recursive implementation, see equations 3.2 and 3.3, the WFLC can be used online to obtain estimations of both tremor frequency and amplitude, [107].

$$w_{0_{k+1}} = w_{0_k} + 2\mu_0 \varepsilon_k \sum_{r=1}^{M} r \left(w_{r_k} x_{M+r_k} - w_{M+r_k} x_{r_k} \right) \tag{3.2}$$

where,

$$x_{rk} = \begin{cases} \sin(r\omega_0 k), & 1 \leq r \leq M \\ \cos((r-M)\omega_0 k), & M+1 \leq r \leq 2M \end{cases} \tag{3.3}$$

Figure 3.1 illustrates the architecture of the WFLC algorithm.

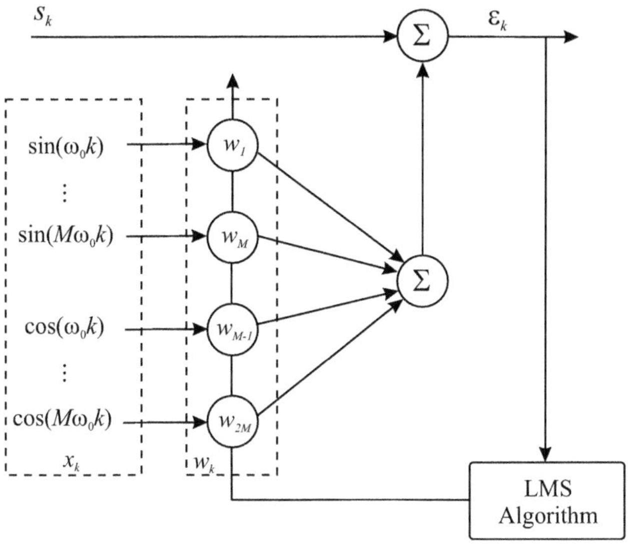

Fig. 3.1 Weighted Fourier Linear Combiner (WFLC) algorithm. The system performs a recursive estimation of the input signal frequency, ω_0. The valued of the harmonics in sines and cosines (x_k vector) are calculated. These values are multiplied by the Foutir coefficients (w_k) and summed in order to obtain the amplitude of the input signal, s_k.

The WFLC algorithm was evaluated with the signals measured in the experiments decribed in previous chapter. In the completed trials, the algorithm was able to estimate the tremor movement of all the patients with accuracy always lower than 2 degrees, see figure 3.2. The main disadvantage of the WFLC is the need for a preliminary filtering stage to eliminate the voluntary component of the movement, [107]. This filtering stage introduces an undesired time lag for our system when estimating tremor movement, this time lag introduces a time delay that could considerably affect the implementation of the control strategies for tremor suppression.

The performance of the algorithm in tracking the tremor frequency in real-time was also evaluated. Figure 3.3 illustrates the behavior of the WFLC for the real-time estimation of tremor frequency for different values of initial frequency, ω_0. Notice that the convergence time to the estimation of the frequency is small for the different initial parameters, figures 3.3c), d), and e). Figure 3.3a) illustrates the patient movement and the WFLC estimation of tremor amplitude, T_{ref}.

3.2 Estimation of Voluntary Movement

As described in the introduction of this chapter, the tremor literature indicates that voluntary movements and tremor movements are considerably different, [33, 80, 107, 108]. Voluntary movements are slower while tremor movements are brusquer. This indicates that adaptive algorithms to estimate and track movement would be

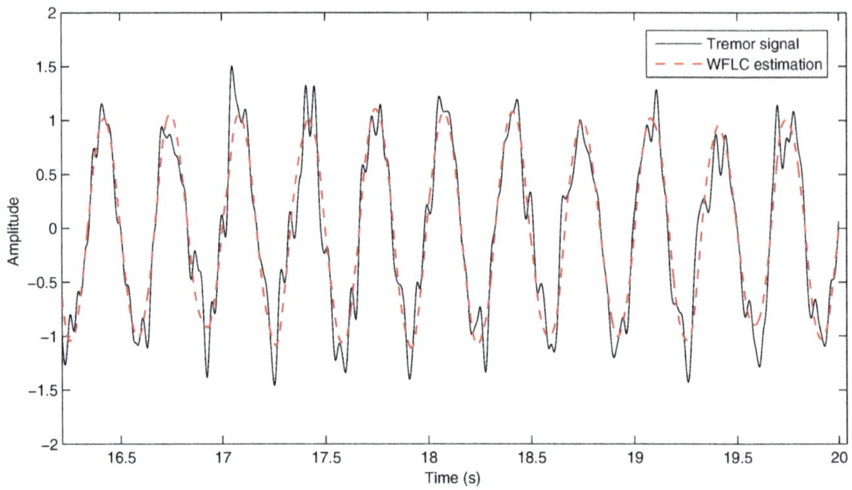

Fig. 3.2 Estimation of tremor, solid line, based on WFLC algorithm, red dashed line.

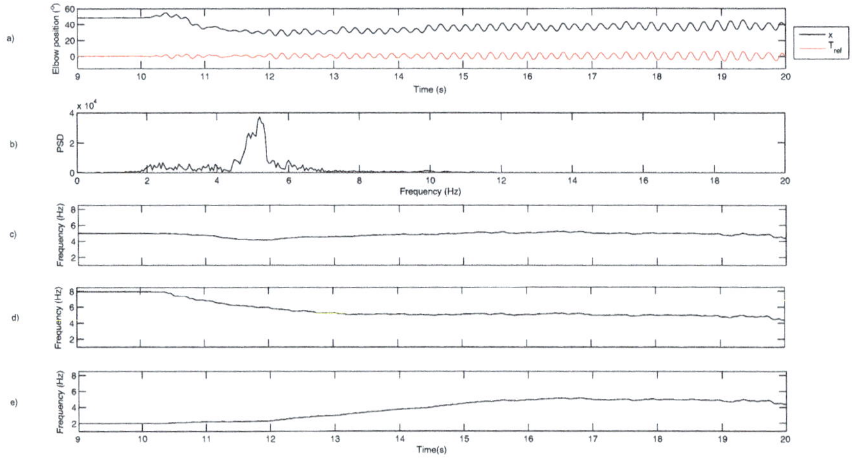

Fig. 3.3 Illustration of the WFLC algorithm performance during the estimation of the tremorous frequency of a patient with Essential tremor. a) x represents the patient movement and T_{ref} the estimation of tremor amplitude, b) Power Density Spectrum of x, notice that patient presents a postural tremor at 5,6 Hz. The initial frequency of the WFLC, ω_0, is different in each trial : c) 8 Hz d) 5 Hz y e) 2 Hz.

useful when separating the two movements with an appropriate design. The underlying idea is to design the filters so that they only estimate the less dynamic component of the input signal, which in our case we consider to be voluntary movement, thereby filtering out the tremor movement.

A set of algorithms was considered for the estimation of the voluntary motion: two point-extrapolator, critically damped g-h estimator, Benedict-Bordner g-h estimator, and Kalman filter. These algorithms implement both estimation and filtering equations. The combination of these actions allows the algorithm to filter out the tremorous movement from the overall motion at the same time it reduces the phase lag introduced, [10]. The equation parameters were adjusted to track the movements with lower dynamics (voluntary movement) since tremors present a behaviour characterised by quick movements.

The algorithms evaluated were two degrees of freedom estimators i.e., they assume a constant velocity movement model. This assumption is reasonable since the sample period is very small compared to the movement velocities, [19], i.e., the sample period adopted was 1 ms and the voluntary movement estimated occurs in a bandwidth lower than 2 Hz. The performance of these algorithms were compared based on their accuracy when estimating voluntary movements of tremor time series from patients.

3.2.1 *Two Points Extrapolator*

It is the simplest tracking algorithm. This algorithm uses the current position measured, y_n, and the past measured position, y_{n-1}, to estimate the velocity, $\dot{x}_n^*$, and the future position x_{n+1}^*.

$$\dot{x}_n^* = \frac{y_n - Y_{n-1}}{T}, \tag{3.4}$$

$$x_{n+1}^* = y_n + T * \dot{x}_n^*, \tag{3.5}$$

where T is the sample time and "$*$" denotes an estimated value.

3.2.2 *g-h Filters*

gh filters are simple recursive filters that estimate the future position and velocity of a variable based on constant velocity dynamic model. Measurements are used to correct these predictions, minimizing the estimation error. gh trackers have been traditionally employed in radar tracking and aeronautics, [19].

Despite of assuming zero acceleration, they provide good performance when this assumption is not fully satisfied. If a Taylor expansion of the state variable x is considered, it is proven that the influence of acceleration $\ddot{x}$ can be neglected if either the sampling period T_s or the acceleration $\ddot{x}$ itself are small. In our case, the sampling period, T_s is 1 ms, which can be considered small, [19]. Also the second derivative of the state variable x, which represents the angular velocity of the voluntary motion, has a maximum 4 orders of magnitude smaller than the average angular velocity. Thus, both assumptions for considering a constant velocity model hold.

The equations of the general gh tracker are:

$$x_{k,k} = x_{k,k-1} + g_k(y_k - x_{k,k-1}) \tag{3.6}$$

$$\dot{x}_{k,k} = \dot{x}_{k,k-1} + \frac{h_k}{T_s}(y_k - x_{k,k-1}) \tag{3.7}$$

$$x_{k+1,k} = x_{k,k} + T_s\dot{x}_{k,k} \tag{3.8}$$

$$\dot{x}_{k+1,k} = \dot{x}_{k,k} \tag{3.9}$$

Equations 3.6 and 3.7 are known as update, tracking or filtering equations. They estimate the current position and velocity of a variable, $x_{k,k}$, $\dot{x}_{k,k}$, based on previous predicted position and velocity, $x_{k,k?1}$, $\dot{x}_{k,k?1}$, having current measurement y_k into account. Confidence on the measures is weighted by the gains g_k and h_k. Equations 3.8 and 3.9 are called prediction equations because they provide a prediction of future position and velocity, $x_{k+1,k}$, $\dot{x}_{k+1,k}$,based on the first order dynamic model of the variable.

gh filters are affected by two error sources, [19]. The lag, dynamic, bias or systematic error, which is related to the constant velocity assumption, and the measurement error, which is inherent to the sensor and measurement process. Both error sources can be put down into g_k and h_k functions form. Typically the smaller g_k and h_k are, the larger is the dynamic error and the smaller are the measurement errors. Therefore, in designing a gh tracking filter there is a degree of freedom in choice of the magnitude of the measurement error relative to the dynamic error. To simplify the selection of gains two filters that are optimal in some sense are considered. These filters are described next.

3.2.2.1 Critically Damped g-h Estimator

The Critical Dampened Filter is an optimal gh tracker based on finding the least-squares fitting line of the previous measurements, [19]. This estimation algorithm does not rely on a traditional least-squares fitting because this would cause old data to be considered as important as latest data. To eliminate this problem, old data is given lesser significance when formulating the total error by weighting them by a factor θ less than one, when forming the total sum:

$$e = \sum_{k=0}^{N} \theta^k (x_k^* - y_k)^2 \tag{3.10}$$

This estimation algorithm is a g-h filter composed by g-h track update equations and by g-h prediction equations:

$$update \begin{cases} \dot{x}^*_{k,k} = \dot{x}^*_{k,k-1} + h_k \left(\frac{y_k - x^*_{k,k-1}}{T} \right) \\ x^*_{k,k} = x^*_{k,k-1} + g_k \left(y_k - x^*_{k,k-1} \right) \end{cases} \tag{3.11}$$

$$predict \begin{cases} \dot{x}^*_{k+1,k} = \dot{x}^*_{k,k} \\ x^*_{k+1,k} = x^*_{k,k} + T\dot{x}^*_{k+1,k} \end{cases} \tag{3.12}$$

The track update equations or estimation equations, 3.11, provide us the velocity and position of tremor at time kT after the measurement of the angular position of the joint, y_k. The estimated position is based on the use of the actual measurement as well as the past prediction. The estimated state contains all the information we need about the past. As a consequence of filtering, the measured noise is reduced. The predicted position is an estimate of x_{n+1} based on past states and prediction (equation 3.12), and take into account the current measurement by means of updated states.

In order to avoid the need of storing all the past values to find the current error, the optimum discounted least-squares tracking filter can be expressed as a constant gh filter where the parameters are related by, [19]:

$$\begin{aligned} g &= 1 - \theta^2 \\ h &= (1 - \theta)^2 \end{aligned} \tag{3.13}$$

The selection of the g-h parameters depends of the dynamics of the target to be tracked and the accuracy desired, [19]. Figures 3.4 and 3.5 illustrate the performance of the Critically damped filter when estimating the voluntary movement (VM_{cd}) of a patient with Essential and Parkinsonian tremor, respectively, when performing the draw a spiral task.

3.2.2.2 Benedict-Bordner g-h Estimator

This estimation algorithm have the same equations that the Critically Damped g-h estimator but with different values in the parameters g-h, [19]. The Benedict-Bordner estimator is designed to minimize the transient error. defined as the weighted sum of the total transient error and the variance of the prediction error due to measurement noise errors, [14]. As a result, it responds faster to changes in target velocity and it's slightly under-damped. Unexpectedly, the filter from this wide class minimizing the total transient error is the constant gh filter that satisfies:

$$h = \frac{g^2}{2 - g} \tag{3.14}$$

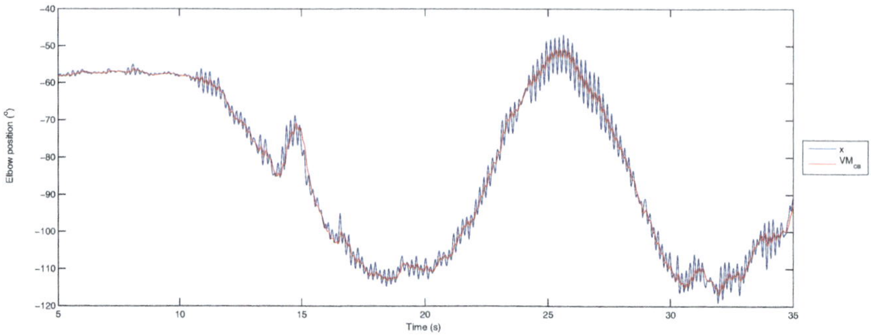

Fig. 3.4 Example of elbow voluntary movement estimation (VM_{cd}) of a patient with Essential tremor while performing the task of draw a spiral (x). The algorithm for estimation was the Critically damped filter. Notice that the delay introduced in the estimation is minimum.

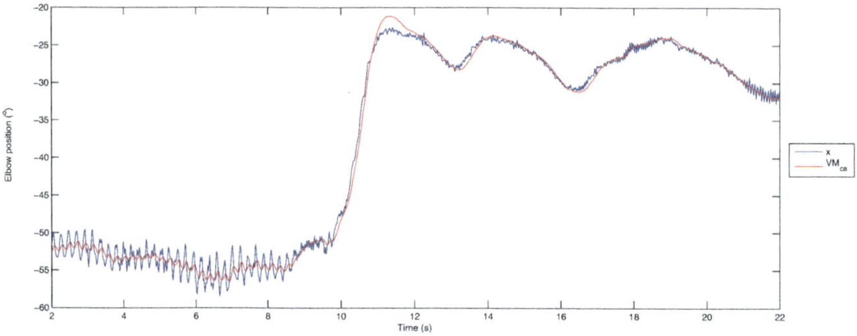

Fig. 3.5 Example of elbow voluntary movement estimation (VM_{cd}) of a patient with Parkinsonian tremor while performing the task of draw a spiral (x). The algorithm for estimation was the Critically damped filter. Notice that the delay introduced in the estimation is minimum.

Therefore, as 3.14 relates g and h, the Benedict-Bordnermfilter has only one degree of freedom to be chosen. As in gh filters increasing the value of $g(h)$ diminishes the transient error, the larger $g(h)$ is, the higher frequencies this algorithm tracks, because it decreases monotonically the dynamic error. Thus, the adequate value of g should track frequencies below 2 Hz still providing good transient response. Figures 3.6 illustrates the performance of the Benedict-bordner filter when estimating the voluntary movement (VM_{bb}) of a patient with Essential tremor when performing the draw a spiral task.

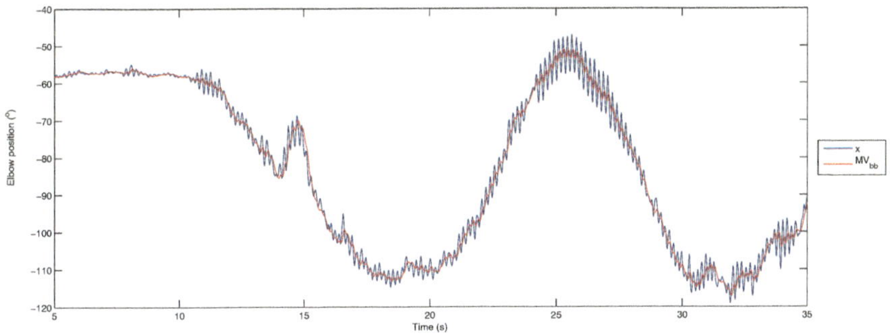

Fig. 3.6 Example of elbow voluntary movement estimation (MV_{bb}) of a patient with Essential tremor while performing the task of draw a spiral (x). The algorithm for estimation was the Benedict-Bordner filter. Notice that the delay introduced in the estimation is minimum.

3.2.3 The Kalman Filter

The Kalman Filter is the most extended estimation algorithm in engineering. It is a recursive linear estimator that successively calculates an estimate for a state that evolves over time, on the basis of periodic observations of this state. It is a g-h filter where the weights g and h are a function of n and are updated recursively. This filter has the advantage of allowing the optimum use of the information if it is available. In addition, permits the use of the target dynamics information to optimize the filter parameters. More complete information about Kalman filter can be found in [10, 18, 19, 66].

In our case, the KF will be used for the same purpose than gh tracking filters, i.e. to estimate voluntary motion ignoring faster tremorous movement. In this context, prediction equation becomes (9). The state vector $x(t)$ is composed by the variable to be estimated, i.e. velocity of the voluntary component of motion, and its derivative. Acceleration (second derivative of $x(t)$) is not considered because its effects can be neglected.

$$\hat{x}_{k,k-1} = \begin{bmatrix} 1 & T \\ 0 & 1 \end{bmatrix} \hat{x}_{k-1,k-1} \tag{3.15}$$

On the other hand, in order to obtain prediction equations, the following equation was defined:

$$H(k) = [1 \ 0] \tag{3.16}$$

The only matrices left to be defined are covariance matrices $Q(k)$ and $R(k)$. As we aim at tracking voluntary motion, it is assumed that tremor is just sensor noise, thus the variance of the tremorous motion can be used to tune the measurement noise covariance $R(k)$. It is also hypothesized that process noise is related to voluntary motion velocity changes due to tremor. A piecewise constant white acceleration

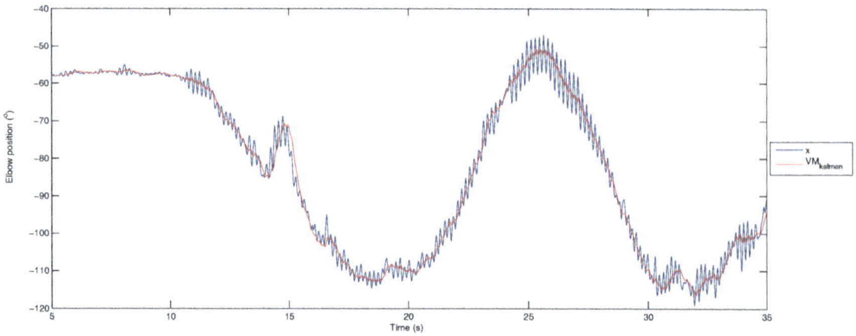

Fig. 3.7 Example of elbow voluntary movement estimation (MV_{kalman}) of a patient with Essential tremor while performing the task of draw a spiral (x). The algorithm for estimation was the Kalman filter.

model is considered, [10]. This model assumes that voluntary motion undergoes constant and uncorrelated acceleration changes between samples, equation 3.17. σ_v^2 is the variance of the random velocity component.

$$R = \sigma_\omega^2 \tag{3.17}$$

$$Q_k = \sigma_v^2 \begin{bmatrix} \frac{T^4}{4} & \frac{T^3}{2} \\ \frac{T^3}{2} & T^2 \end{bmatrix} \tag{3.18}$$

In order to select the values for the parameters σ_v^2 and σ_ω^2 that characterize the covariance matrices, i.e. measurement and process noise, the recorded data is examined. Measurement Noise, σ_ω^2, is modelled as the average covariance of the isolated tremor, $\sigma_\omega^2 = 0.0643\ \frac{rad^2}{s^{-2}}$. The value of σ_v^2 that defines process noise is sought within the $0.5\max_{\ddot{x}} \leq |\sigma_v| \leq \max_{\ddot{x}}$ interval as recommended in [10]. Calculating the second derivative of the recorded motion, the maximum of the acceleration is obtained, $\max_{\ddot{x}} = 0.1042\ \frac{rad}{s^{-3}}$.

Figures 3.7 and 3.8 illustrate the performance of the Kalman filter when estimating the voluntary movement (VM_{kalman}) of a patient with Essential and Parkinsonian tremor, respectively, when performing the draw a spiral task. Kalman filter, as expected, provides almost the same absolute estimation error for different covariance matrices (if they are chosen in the adequate interval) because it continuously adapts its gain to minimize the a posteriori estimation error. Thus, small deviations in the parameters are compensated by the filter itself. The only noticeable difference is the settling time at the beginning of the estimation. The KF provides the lowest absolute error among the candidate algorithms because it is capable of adapting its gain

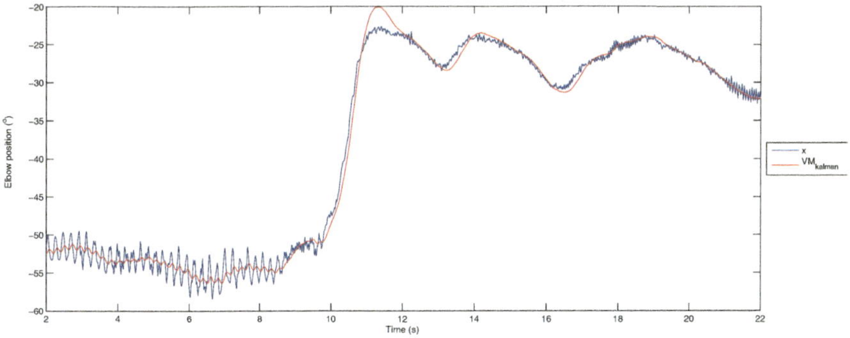

Fig. 3.8 Example of elbow voluntary movement estimation (MV_{kalman}) of a patient with Parkinsonian tremor while performing the task of draw a spiral (x). The algorithm for estimation was the Kalman filter.

to abrupt transients, something that constant gain filters like gh filters can not do. In fact, gh filters are regarded as a steady state filters, because their performance degrades during transient periods, [10].

3.2.4 Figure of Merit

In order to quantitative compare the estimators proposed a metric, *Cinematic Estimation Error (CEE)*, was proposed. The equation that define this metrics is:

$$CEE = \sqrt{\varphi^2_{|b^*|} + \sigma^2_{x^*}}, \tag{3.19}$$

where $\varphi^2_{|b^*|}$ is the mean square of errors of the estimators: $|b^*| = |x_k - x^*_{k,k-1}|$, and $\sigma^2_{x^*}$ variance of the estimation.

CEE quantifies the transient response through $\varphi^2_{|b^*|}$ and, at the same time, the averaging or filtering capabilities of the filter through the term $\sigma^2_{x^*}$. The accuracy and transient response of the estimation algorithms are important. Another important parameter taken into account in our analysis was the execution time of each algorithm in view of the fact that the system was designed to work in real time.

Comparing the performance of the candidate filters for the above selected parameter, it was observed that Benedict-Bordner filter presents the best results with the lowest computational cost. The metrics indicated that Kalman filter has a performance slight better than Benedict-Bordner filter but its computational cost is higher. As realtime estimation and computational burden are a major consideration in this

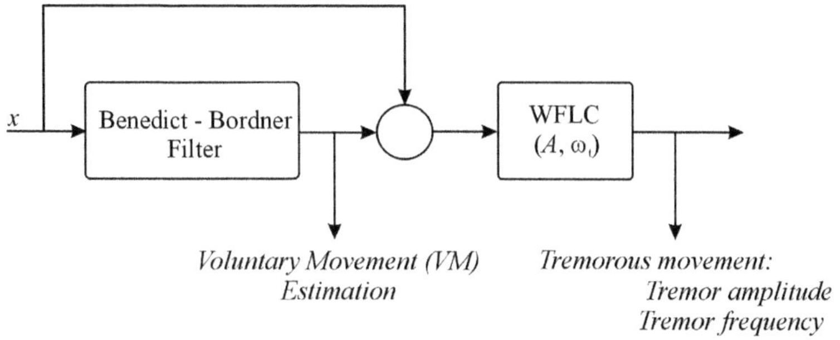

Fig. 3.9 Two-stage tremor modelling: first, the low frequency content voluntary motion is estimated, secondly, the voluntary motion estimation is subtracted from the original motion, eventually, tremor frequency and amplitude are determined.

work, Benedict-Bordner filter was selected as the best voluntary motion estimation algorithm.

3.3 Real-Time Estimation of Voluntary and Tremorous Movement

The solution adopted was the development of an algorithm capable of estimating voluntary and tremorous motion with a small phase lag based on a two-stage algorithm, see figure 3.9.

In the first stage, the Benedict-Bordner filter estimates the voluntary component of the movements. In the second stage, the estimated voluntary motion is removed from the overall motion and it is assumed that the remaining movement is tremor. After this, the WFLC was used in order to estimate tremor parameters. In this stage, the algorithm estimates both the amplitude and the time-varying frequency of the tremorous movement.

The algorithm proposed was evaluated with data obtained from the patients measured during the experiments presented in the previous chapter. The estimation error of the first stage was 1.4 ± 1.3 degrees. The second stage algorithm has a convergence time always smaller than 2 s for all signals evaluated and the Mean Square Error (MSE) between the estimated tremor and the *real tremor* (obtained off-line by means of manual decomposition based on classical filter techniques), after the convergence, is smaller than 1 degree. The combination of both techniques resulted in a very efficient algorithm with small processing cost for estimating in real time the voluntary and the tremorous components of the overall motion, [113]. Figure 3.10 illustrates the performance of the algorithm when splitting voluntary and tremorous movements of a patient of essential tremor.

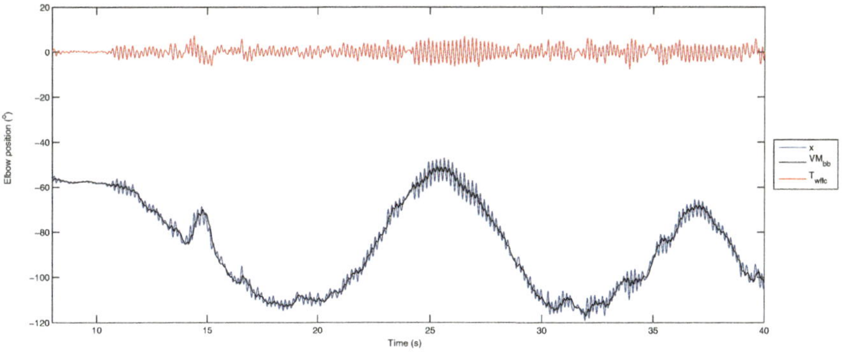

Fig. 3.10 Performance of the two-stage algorithm proposed in order to distinguish in real-time voluntary movement from tremor. The movement (x) corresponds to the elbow joint of a patient with Essential tremor while performing the task draw a spiral. Notice that the algorithm is composed by two stages, the first estimates the voluntary movement by means of a Benedict-Bordner filter (VMbb), the second stage is responsible for estimating the tremorous movement (Twflc) by using the WFLC algorithm.

3.4 Conclusions

In this chapter a two-stage algorithm for realtime estimation of tremor amplitude and frequency based on IMU information is presented and validated. Quantification of instantaneous tremor parameters plays an important role in three domains of application. First, clinical scales and diagnostic criteria rely on tremor frequency as the only objectively measurable feature. Second, neuroscientists measure and model upper limb oscillations to employ them as a window to investigate central and peripheral mechanisms that underly motor control and tremor pathogenesis. Finally, and most important in the context of this book, robotics based tremor management techniques require adequate tremor models in order to efficiently exploit the possibilities of biomechanical loading.

The algorithm developed presents the following advantages for its application in ambulatory devices for tremor suppression: a) Estimate the voluntary movement, b) Estimate the tremorous movement, c) The delay introduced for the estimation is 1ms and the convergence time is always smaller than 2 s, d) Estimate both the amplitude and the frequency of the tremorous movement, e) Presents a low computation cost.

Chapter 4
Upper Limb Exoskeleton for Tremor Suppression: Physical HR Interaction

The scientific and medical community is becoming more and more interested in the so-called Rehabilitation Robotics. Rehabilitation Robotics has been envisioned as technology for the restoration and functional compensation of people suffering from physical disability or disorders, either for the rehabilitation therapy or assistance of people.

In robotic field, exoskeletons are mechatronic devices of which segments and joints correspond to some extend to these of the human body and the system is externally coupled to the person (wearable robot). The primary applications of exoskeletons were teleoperation and power amplification. Later, exoskeletons have been considered as devices for rehabilitation and assistance of disabled or elderly people by means of upper and/or lower limb orthosis. Lastly, taking into account that robotic exoskeletons are able to apply independent dynamic forces on human joints and segments, these devices permits to realize experiments and studies on motor control, adaptation and neuro-motor research.

One important and specific aspect in Rehabilitation Robotics is the intrinsic interaction between human and robot. This interaction is twofold. First, cognitive, because the human controls the robot while it provides feedback to the human; second, a biomechanical interaction leading to the application of controlled forces between both actors. There is a physical interface between person and device to provide the mechanical power. Concerns of this physical interface are safety, robustness and reliability of the robotic mechanism taking into account the characteristics of the human neuromuscular-skeletal system.

This chapter is focused on describing in detail the development of the upper limb exoskeleton WOTAS (Wearable Orthosis for Tremor Assessment and Suppression). In the framework of the DRIFTS (Dynamically Responsive Intervention For Tremor Suppression) project, [81], the WOTAS exoskeleton was presented with two main objectives: monitoring and diagnosis, and validation of non-grounded tremor reduction strategies, [115].

Moreover, two novel nongrounded control strategies for suppression of tremor by means of an orthotic (wearable) exoskeleton are presented. Both are based on biomechanical loading, but one is active while the other is passive. 1) Tremor

E. Rocon and J.L. Pons: Exoskeletons in Rehabilitation Robotics, STAR 69, pp. 67–98.
springerlink.com

reduction through impedance control. This strategy modifies the stiffness, damping and mass properties of the upper limb in order to suppress tremor. 2) Notch filtering at tremor frequency. This strategy implements an active noise filter at the tremor frequency taking advantage of the repetitive characteristics of tremor.

4.1 Biomechanics of the Upper Limb

Cancelling tremor by mechanical loading the upper limb by robotic exoskeletons implies an inherent physical interaction between user and robot. There are two main concerns regarding the biomechanics of this interaction:

1. The user's tolerance to pressure
2. Mechanical characterization of the soft tissues of the upper-limb

4.1.1 Tolerance to Pressure

The *Pressure distribution* is one of the main concerns related to the orthotics field. The most important function of any orthotic device is related to load transmission to the body bony structures through the soft tissues. Therefore, there are several factors in relation with pressure that have to be taken into account, namely, safety, pain and comfort.

There are two basic strategies to manage an external load: concentrate loads over a small region with high tolerance to pressures or distribute the load over an area as big as possible to reduce the pressure. The last approach matches the strategy for preventing pain or injuries, so it is commonly adopted as the right one, but comfort can differ substantially from this approach. For instance, Krooskop et al., [73], have shown that mattresses with uniform pressure distribution can cause restless. Goonetilleke shows in its work that there should be a threshold in which it is better to concentrate than to distribute forces, [45]. The reason for that should be the Spatial Summation Theory that claims that as the area of contact increases the number of excited skin receptors also increases and subsequently the comfort perception is worst. Two main aspects have been analyzed:

1. User perception of pressure
2. pressure threshold for discomfort

A study based on the methodology proposed by Gonzalez et al., [47], was carried out in order to find-out the Pressure Discomfort Threshold (PDT). In the afore mentioned study, the methodology was applied to foot pressure distribution. Nevertheless, results from this study suggested that the methodology could be appropriate to analyze the ability to support pressure in the upper limb.

Pressure discomfort threshold has been studied in nine subjects, all of them affected by tremor at the upper limb. The mean age was 53.67 years old (std. dev. 21.01). Measurement points have been located taking into account the common placement of load transmission elements of upper-limb tremor suppression orthoses.

These points were chosen on the dorsal and palmar side, over muscles and over bony areas in order to have a good representation of the different areas of the forearm. We used a dynamometer for measurements. The indentor was an aluminum cylindrical cap with a contact flat surface of 1.3 cm^2 adapted to the dynamometer. Pressure was applied five times on each point. The sequence of pressure application was randomized previously in order to avoid the learning effect of the patient in each point.

In this study, no significant differences have been found in pressure discomfort threshold between the points analyzed, and therefore no significant differences were found in the pressure sensitivities. Subsequently, there are no preferred locations to fix the orthosis force interface to the upper limb. Whatever point in the forearm can manage the same pressure in relation with comfort. Pressure thresholds pattern are shown in Figure 4.1.

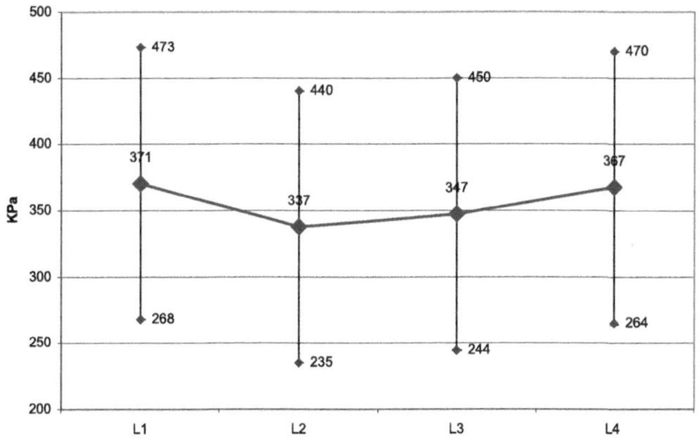

Fig. 4.1 Pressure tolerance threshold pattern.

The maximum pressure for discomfort found in the forearm was 230 KPa. In order to ensure comfort, maximum values should have to be at least one order of magnitude under this figure.

4.1.2 Mechanical Characterization of Soft Tissues at the Upper-Limb

Stiffness between the orthotic device and the body is a key factor to take into account in order to control a dynamic process such as tremor. The exoskeleton must transmit the loads to the bones for tremor suppression. This transmission is mediated by the soft tissues between the supports and the actuator. Usually, the effect of load transmission is negligible in common orthotics. However, tremor has a pure dynamic component. Therefore the characteristics of the transmissions through the soft tissues will play an important role in the efficiency of tremor suppression. The soft tissues involved in the transmission are basically skin, fat and tendons for the hand and skin, fat and muscles for the forearm.

The mechanical characteristics of soft tissues is highly non-linear, [88], and can vary deeply from one user to other (for instance with the presence of oedema) or can change dynamically (i.e. the stiffness of muscles varies deeply as the muscles are contracting). The equivalent stiffness of the tissue increases as the stress increases. A strain-stress curve for soft tissues is represented in Figure 4.2. As it can be seen, the curve is characterized by an hysteresis. In our first approach, since the orthotic devices are attached once and then they have slow movements from this position, just the rising part of the stress curve was considered.

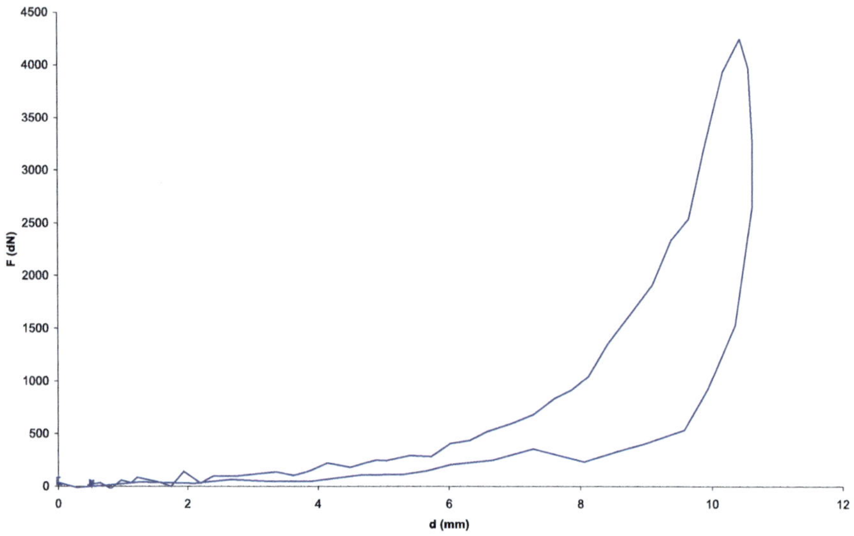

Fig. 4.2 Strain stress curve for the forearm.

A study to characterize the soft tissues at different points of the upper limb has been performed. Measurement points have been located taking into account the common placement of load transmission elements of upper-limb orthoses. According to our study, no major differences related to gender could be found. It was also concluded that the soft tissues of the forearm could be modeled by a third degree polynomial that describes the deformation of the tissue according to the force applied.

Other factors were studied, such as the effects of age in in the stress-strain characteristics. Nevertheless, it was concluded that the differences on the skin mechanical behavior could be ignored since its effects are much lower than others factors, for instance the obesity, [5].

4.2 Wearable Orthosis for Tremor Assessment and Suppression, WOTAS

An orthosis is defined as a medical device that acts in parallel to a segment of the body in order to compensate some dysfunction. The upper limb main function is to guarantee that the hand realizes its functions and can reach any point in the space, specially any point in human surface, in such a way, that the person can manipulate, draw on, and move objects, from or to the body. Therefore, the kinematic chain formed by the shoulder, elbow, forearm, wrist, and hand, has a high mobility degree, and a high prehension capacity with an infinite number of positions and functions. The upper limb is one of the most anatomic and physiologically complex part of the body.

The upper limb is very important because it is able to execute cognitive-driven, expression-driven, and manipulation activities. Furthermore, it intervenes in the exploration of the environment and in all reflex motor acts. Then, any alteration or pathology that affects the upper limb motion range, muscle power, sensibility, skin integrity, will alter its operation. The concept of WOTAS is to develop an active upper limb exoskeleton based on robotics technologies capable of applying forces to cancel tremor and retrieving kinematic information from the upper limb.

4.2.1 Mechanical Design

The WOTAS concept will provide a means of testing non-grounded tremor reduction strategies. WOTAS follows the kinematic structure of the human upper limb and spans the elbow an wrist joints, see figure 4.8. It exhibits three degrees of freedom corresponding to elbow flexion-extension, forearm pronation-supination and wrist flexion extension.In the final design, WOTAS restricts the movement of wrist adduction-abduction, nevertheless this movement is the less functional movement in the upper limb, [6]. Furthermore, as in WOTAS fingers remain free and wrist abduction-adduction is dependent to the finger movements, [67], the functional reduction is even lesser.

The mechanical design of the joints for elbow flexion-extension, and wrist flexion-extension are similar to other orthotic solutions and are based in the behavior of those physiological joints as hinges. For orthotic purposes, flexion-extension movement is considered as a pure rotational movement. Therefore, this axis of rotation should be used for the rotational actuator. The axis of rotation for the elbow joint is placed in the line between the two epicondyles. The axis of rotation for the wrist joint is located in the line between the capital and lunate bones of the carpus.

The mechanical design for the control of the pronation supination movement is more complex and it is explained below.

4.2.1.1 Pronation-Supination Control

The pronation-supination movement of the forearm is a rotational movement of the forearm on its longitudinal axis which engages two joints that are mechanically connected: the upper radioulnar joint (which belongs to the elbow) and the lower radioulnar joint (which belongs to the wrist), [67]. There are two bones in the forearm that make this movement possible:

- The ulna is the bone that remains fixed during the pronation-supination movement. It constitutes the main part of the elbow, in particular the olecranon.
- The radius is the moving bone in the pronation and supination. It rotates in proximal part (close to the elbow) and moves distally along the axis formed by the ulna bone (see figure 4.3).

Both bones have a shape approximately pyramidal and they are placed in such a way that the base of the radius is in the tip of the ulna and vice-versa.

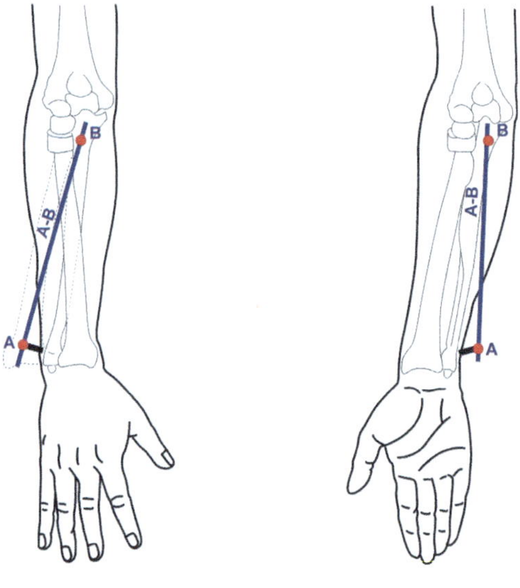

Fig. 4.3 Scheme of the pronation-supination control.

The WOTAS platform controls the pronation-supination movement with the rotation control of a bar parallel to the forearm. This bar is fixed very close to the olecranon (point B, figure 4.3). Thus the bar is fixed to the ulnar position at elbow level. The distal fixation of the bar is made at the head of the radius, although the bar is maintained in the ulnar side in order to minimize the excursion of the system. This fixation is explained later in the support design section.

4.2.1.2 Design of the Support System

There are no static orthoses that achieve tremor suppression due to the intrinsically dynamics characteristics of tremor. In these cases, the tremor suppression mechanism tends to lose their alignment instead of suppressing tremor.

To determine the points of the upper limb where the dynamic forces would be applied, i.e, the points where the arm supports would be placed for the interface between the actuators and the arm, a number of biomechanical and physiological considerations of the upper limb have to be observed, such as [95]: 1) the forces on the arm tissues must stay in acceptable limits 2) the application of forces on the arm that have minimal interference of elbow and wrist movement 3) the interaction of the robotic device with the arm, i.e., where the forces will be applied on the upper limb and how the load will be transmitted to the person for optimum comfort. Joint movements areas, bony prominences, surface tendons and surface nerves or vessels should be avoided.

To respond to these issues a biomechanical study was done of the upper limb, [95]. The aim of this study was to determine the limits of comfort regarding pressure, so that there is an upper limit to the total force that can be applied safely to the upper limb, see figure 4.4. This study analysed two key aspects: the person's perception of the pressure and the maximum pressure tolerance thresholds. The first aspect is important to select the appropriate strategy to apply to the load on the body.

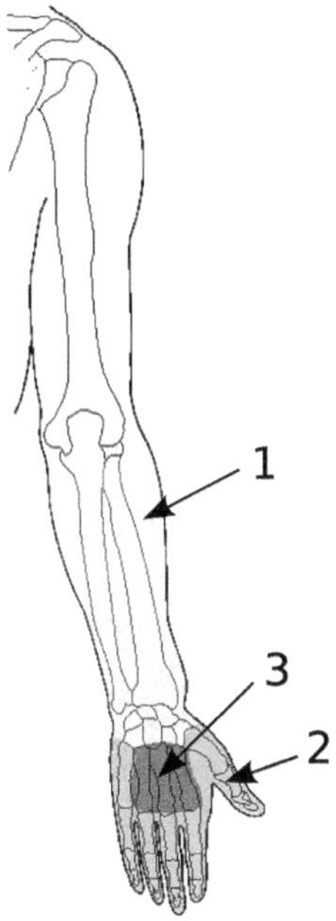

Fig. 4.4 Areas of sensitivity to pressure in the hand and forearm: (1) Low-tolerance area (average ca. 450 kPa), (2) Middle-tolerance are and (3) High-tolerance area (average ca. 950 kPa).

For the development of the mechanical structure, different types of materials for the securing or support elements between the orthotic device and the arm were considered. The mechanical conditions of these elements are critical because they must ergonomically couple the upper limb, and also the rigidity of the material must be greater than the rigidity of the underlying tissues. To securely fix the structure it was decided to use supports made from thermoplastic. With this type of material, supports are obtained that adapt to the morphology of each user's arm, figure 4.5. Each support has at least three contact points per segment and thus misalignments are avoided between the orthosis and limb. Velcro straps were fixed to the fabric in order to tighten the support to the arm. The fixation to the wrist is mainly placed over the radial side for the reason that the wrist follows the movement of the head of the radius. Both the distal tip of the pronation-supination control and the proximal tip of the wrist control are fixed to the ulnar side of the wrist. The fixation to the hand is very similar to that of the wrist. In addition, a textile substrate was used to compress the soft tissues and enhance performance of the fixation supports.

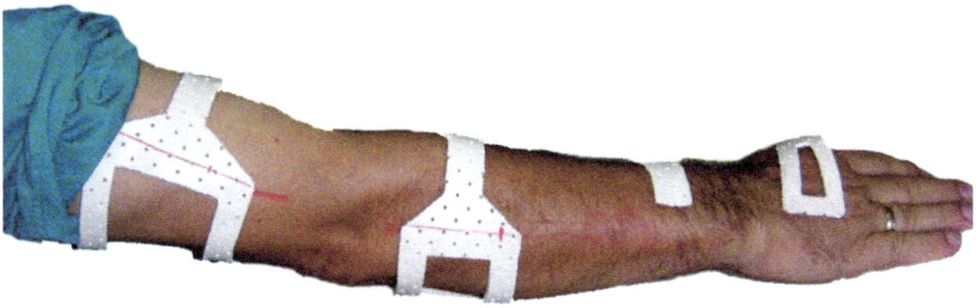

Fig. 4.5 Structure of WOTAS support.

4.2.2 *Sensors*

The system aims to allow both monitoring of tremor data and implementation of tremor suppression strategies. Therefore, it is equipped with kinematic (angular velocity) and kinetic (interaction force between limb and orthosis) sensors.

Tremor force, position, velocity and acceleration are the required information to implement the two control strategies. The types of sensors were restricted to the following sensors: goniometry, gyroscopes and accelerometers. MEMS gyroscopes were selected as a promising technology. The main advantages of using gyroscopes were described in section 2.4.1.1.

4.2.2.1 Force Sensors

Since no backdrivable actuators were chosen for the application (see next section), it was also decided to use force sensors as a means of implementing impedance feedback control strategies. Strain gauges in a full Wheatstone bridge have been selected as force sensors. The gauges measure the torque applied by the motors on the WOTAS structure, therefore, they are mounted on the structure so that they only measure the force perpendicular to the motor axis (F_m), thus their measurement is not affected by forces caused in undesired directions, figure 4.6. The extensiometric gauges are connected to a Wheatstone Bridge circuit in a combination of four active gauges (full bridge).

The strain gauge system was characterized and the sensitivities of the system were derived in the three planes. The tests performed showed that the system has a very low sensitivity to orthogonal forces. The system presented a thermal drift, however, after a few minutes the output voltage becomes stable and suitable for operation.

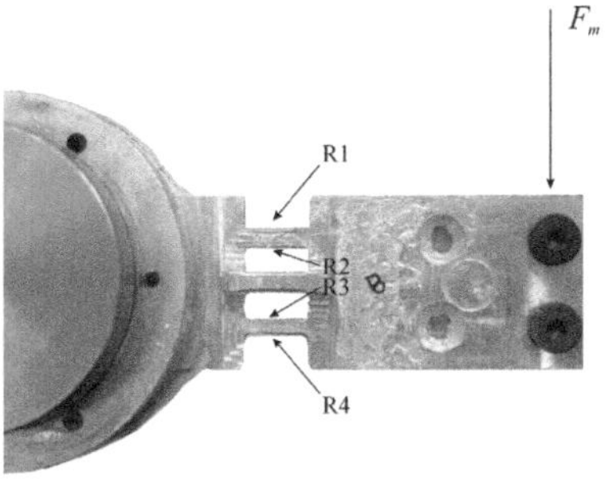

Fig. 4.6 Full Wheatstone bridge and gauges (R1, R2, R3, R4) mounted on WOTAS structure.

4.2.3 Actuators

Before the selection of specific actuators to suppress tremor, an estimation of the required torque and power was performed. This was achieved through an analysis of kinematic tremor data presented in section 2.4.4 . From this torque estimation of effort that the exoskeleton structure must support, duralumin was selected as the material to construct the exoskeleton structure. This material was selected in order to build a lightweight structure with sufficient rigidity to support the efforts.

Based on this study, a number of candidate actuators were evaluated, [115]. The analysis was restricted to the following actuators: Electro Active Polymers (EAPs), Electro and Magneto Rheological fluids (ERF-MRF), DC motors, Shape Memory Actuators (SMAs), Pneumatic muscles and Ultrasonic Motors.

The actuator technology should have a high power density allowing the implementation of a compact and light solution suitable for wearable devices. Based on this criteria both DC motors and Ultrasonic motors can be regarded as best alternatives for exerting tremor suppression forces. The former are well-known off the-shelf technologies of easy integration in advanced control schemes but bulky. The latter are less flexible but offer very compact solutions due to their dynamic range (low velocity high torque motors). Both alternatives were evaluated in prototypes and DC motor was the technology selected for the final version of WOTAS. The main problem with the ultrasonic motors was their poor response at low speed, therefore leading to problems to track user's slow voluntary motion, [109].

Owing to the problems encountered with ultrasonic motors, a new WOTAS device was constructed using DC motors as an actuation element. The DC motor

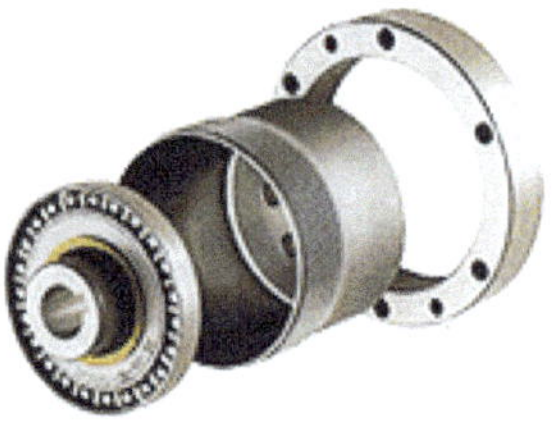

Fig. 4.7 Harmonic Drive HDF-014-100-2A.

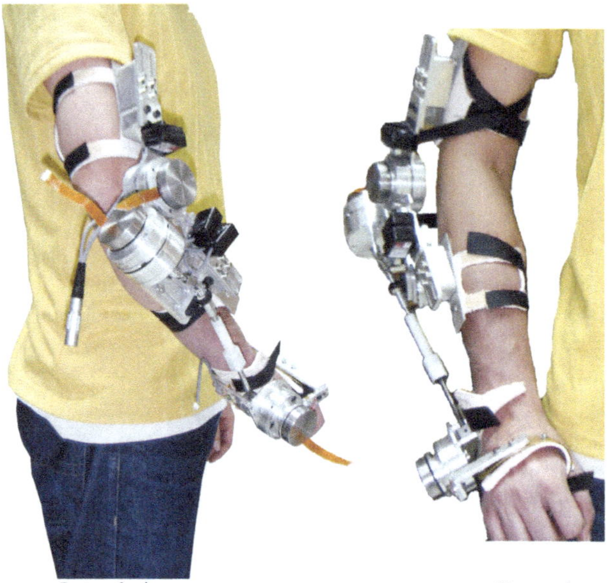

Lateral view Front view

Fig. 4.8 Final version of WOTAS for the control of three human upper-limb movements: flexion-extension of the elbow, flexion-extension of the wrist and pronation-supination of the forearm.

selected to activate WOTAS articulations was a Maxon DC flat brushless motor EC45. In order to match the speed and torque of the DC motor to the application requirements, a harmonic transmission drive was used. In particular, the drive selected for our application was the HDF-014-100-2A, figure 4.7. This configuration, based on flat DC motors and pancake transmissions, is able to provide a maximum torque of 8 N.m, nevertheless the maximum torque was electronically limited to 3 N.m in order to guarantee the safety of the user. Figure 4.8 illustrates the final configuration of WOTAS system activated by DC motors.

The total weight of the final system is roughly 850 g. A protocol for testing the system was performed to evaluate the usability and the range of workspace allowed to a normal user. The system was used in the laboratory to perform a wide variety of manoeuvres in free mode. These preliminary tests successfully showed the correct operation of the system and the capability of the system to access the workspace, without affecting the normal range of motion of the user, [115].

4.3 Control Architecture

The WOTAS control architecture basically consists of 3 components: 1) the exoskeleton, with its structure, sensors and actuators 2) a control unit, responsible for executing the algorithms in real time to suppress the tremor and the acquisition card for the interface between the sensors, actuators and the controller 3) a remote computer, which in our case executes an application developed for the interface between the system and the doctor who is using it. This control strategy is illustrated in figure 4.9.

This control architecture interfaces the control algorithms with the orthosis. The WOTAS circuitry and sensors serve two functions: 1) To obtain the position, angular

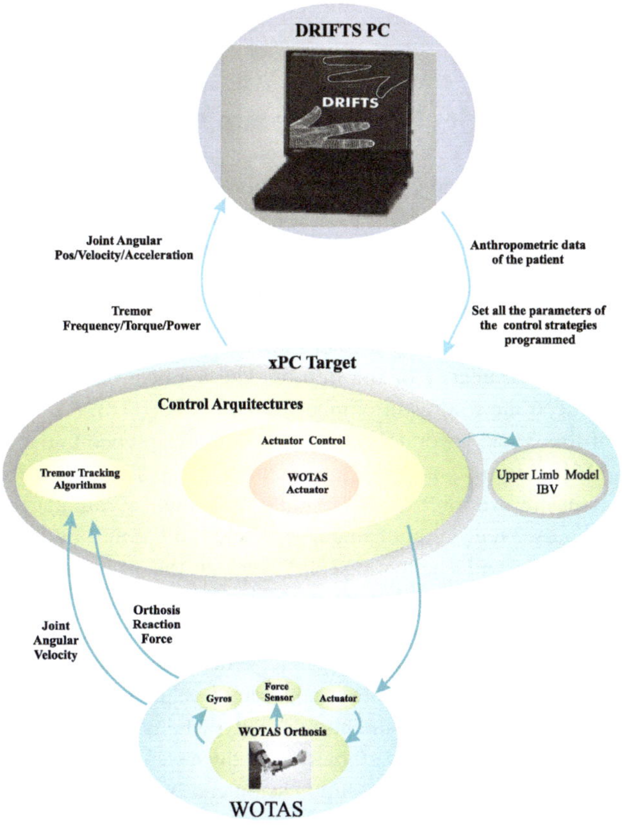

Fig. 4.9 WOTAS control architecture.

velocity and acceleration signals needed for control, data collection and evaluation. 2) To generate the power signal to activate the actuator.

The control of the entire active orthosis was implemented in the MatLab RT environment. This environment provides mathematically complex control strategies in real time. The interface between the MatLab environment and the active orthosis is based on a standard data acquisition board.

In order to provide an interface to all the control strategies a software application was developed in C language. It communicates with the low level controller (either by TPC/IP, wired serial link or BlueTooth) using Dynamic Link Libraries (DLLs) developed by the authors, [115]. This interface monitors signals and tune controller parameters in real time during the control strategy execution. It has five main objectives: 1) Monitoring and validation of algorithms for tremor suppression, 2) Data analysis (statistics, algorithms performance, etc.), 3) Storage of user information such as clinical and anthropometrics data, 4) Comparison between different control strategies., 5) Extraction of user parameters: joint position, velocity and acceleration; tremor frequency (algorithm implemented in the Target PC); tremor torque and power (based on an upper limb biomechanical model).

It was also possible to save all the information retrieved by the sensors for future off-line analysis.

4.4 Control Strategies for Tremor Suppression

Evidence in the literature indicates that applying biomechanical loads on tremor movement reduces its amplitude, [1, 28, 71, 116]. The approach to suppress the pathological tremor within this study is to assist the limb with compensatory technology in order to decrease the amplitude of tremor. The concept of absorbing tremor movement is based on an external device that acts parallel to the upper limb, actively or passively, by applying a load between the limb and a reference point, thereby dissipating the energy of the tremor. The application of inertia, viscosity and friction reduced the tremor in clinical trials, [1, 28, 116]. As was seen in the first chapter of this book, several devices have been developed under this concept, [71, 89, 92, 116]. One of the main drawbacks of the systems described in literature is that the dissipative force is also loading the patient's voluntary motion. As a consequence, the user feels a mechanical resistance to the motion. Even though in adaptive systems this could be avoided, filtering out the voluntary motion we can eliminate the resistance to the voluntary motion.

Applying a biomechanical load to reduce tremor can be done with both portable devices (robotic exoskeletons) and fixed devices (devices mounted on platforms, for example, wheelchairs), [108]. The first approach is characterised by applying internal forces on specific joints of the human body, whereas the second approach is based on applying external forces globally to reduce tremor. Both ambulatory and non-ambulatory concepts for tremor suppression can be found in the literature. As was mentioned in the bibliographical review in chapter 1, there are few ambulatory solutions to reduce tremor. Kotovsky in his studies, [71], established general guidelines for the design of appliances for suppressing tremor which affect the following control strategies:

- Selective reduction of the tremor: robotic exoskeletons must apply a biomechanical load on the upper limb to reduce the tremor without affecting the voluntary movement of the joint.
- The elastic rigidity of the exoskeleton must be minimal so that users do not feel any discomfort in non-neutral positions.
- Safety: so it does not cause any injury to the user while it is being worn.

The general objective to develop control strategies for suppressing tremor with robotic exoskeletons was defined from these design guidelines. Shortly, the control system should work as follows:

1. The exoskeleton sensors measure the tremor movement and interaction force between the exoskeleton and limb in each of the exoskeleton joints. This signal is electronically conditioned for its integration into the control architecture of the exoskeleton.
2. An algorithm (described in previous chapter) discriminates between tremor movement and voluntary movement in real time. Thus biomechanical loads can be selectively applied just on the upper limb to cancel tremor movement. The effect of the tremor cancelling forces on the voluntary movement of the patient is therefore reduced.
3. The information on tremor movement is the input to the controller that will command the actuator responsible for applying forces to cancel the tremor.

This control strategy can be implemented both actively and passively. Passively, a mechanical damper is used, [71], which generates a dissipation force on the tremor movement. It is based on increasing the damping of the biomechanical oscillation system where the tremor is generated. In active systems, [116], actuators generate a movement of equal amplitude but in counter phase from the real-time estimate of the tremor component of movement. Thus the system actively cancels and effectively subtracts the tremor from the total movement of the exoskeleton user. Unlike the passive approach, in which the energy of the tremor movement is dissipated, active systems transfer energy (in counter phase to the tremor movement) to the system.

In accordance with the bibliographical review in this book, the active approach for suppressing tremor has never been implemented in any system for this purpose.

In this chapter control strategies for exoskeletons designed to suppress tremor in the upper-limb joints will be developed. One of the key points in developing exoskeleton control strategies is the intrinsic interaction between the human body and robot. This biomechanical interaction is related to applying controlled dynamic forces between the human and robot. The algorithm controlling the forces applied by the exoskeleton on the limb is responsible for this biomechanical interaction, [51, 54].

The force control of robots that interact with the environment is a field of intense research. PhD theses and articles are regularly published on this issue in magazines and at conferences. This is primarily because of bibliographical contributions in the field of haptic simulation in virtual environments and in that of manipulator robot control. A usual classification in the bibliography, [117], establishes two major approaches for force control: force-position hybrid control ([87, 101]) and impedance control, [54]. In hybrid control, the force in some directions of the robot end and the position of the complementary directions are controlled. Impedance control is based on actively adjusting the mechanical impedance of the system, i.e. the relationship between force, position and its derivatives. It is a generalisation of damping control presented by Whitney, [139], and rigidity control formulated by Salisbury, [119]. As their names indicate, in the first method a relationship is established between the force and velocity magnitudes, whereas in the second the relationship is between the force and position magnitudes. A recent, exhaustive review on the different force-control methods is found in the book by Surdilovic and Vukobratovic, [127].

In rehabilitation robotics, the most commonly used approach to control patient-robot interaction is impedance control, [50, 53]. The basic principles and main considerations on impedance control were established in the excellent work by Hogan, [54, 55, 56]. In his articles, Hogan studies causality conditions in dynamic interaction between a manipulator and the environment. Moreover, Hogan uses the concept of mechanical impedance to model the mechanics of the musculoskeletal system. This study also implements the same approach for robot control. Finally, impedance is selected for a specific application. Hogan thus sets the bases for developing control strategies to control biomechanical interaction between a robotic device and human being.

After an exhaustive bibliographical review of tremor characteristics and control strategies for applying forces on the human body, two control strategies were defined for suppressing tremor with biomechanical loads,[108, 110]:

1. *Tremor reduction through impedance control*: a strategy is defined for controlling impedance of the upper-limb-exoskeleton set. In this instance the rigidity, damping and inertia parameters of the upper limb are altered to study their effects on tremor in the joints of this limb.
2. *Implementation of a notch filter focusing on the frequency of tremor movement.* The use of noise reduction techniques is considered as an alternative to actively suppressing the pathological tremor.

4.4.1 Tremor Reduction through Impedance Control

The impedance of a system can be defined as a relationship between the reaction force of the system to an imposed external motion and the motion itself. In general, impedance comprises three components, i.e. stiffness, damping and inertia. There is evidence, [1], that all three components modify the biomechanical characteristics of tremor at the upper limb.

The approach in this work models the musculoskeletal system (each joint of the upper limb which contributes to the tremor) as a second-order biomechanical system, [1, 92]. It is known that the frequency response of a second-order system behaves like a low-pass filter. The cut-off frequency of this filter is directly related to the biomechanical parameters of the second-order system. The proposed approach consists of selecting the appropriate inertia and damping parameters, so that the cut-off frequency, f_c, of the musculoskeletal system is immediately above the maximum frequency of voluntary movement, cancelling the tremor component of overall movement (see figure 4.10). Unlike other approaches in the literature, the control scheme is conceived so that the effect of the suppression load on voluntary motion is minimized.). In our application the angular position (rigidity control) is not fed back to the system because the position feedback (closed loop) introduces an undesired attenuation in the low-frequency movements, [92]. This attenuation would affect the voluntary movements of the patient and this is an undesired characteristic for our system.

The control architecture proposed in this work is conceived in such a way that the effect on voluntary movement is minimal. One of the major challenges of this approach is separating tremor movement from voluntary movement before applying the correcting action. This requires estimating both movements in real time, as described in chapter 3. The control algorithm depicted in figure 4.11 is the one proposed for altering the biomechanical parameters of the upper limb. As can be observed in the figure, the force control applied by the exoskeleton on the arm is based on admittance control. Thus, the force control applied by the exoskeleton on the arm is implemented with external control loops of the force around an internal velocity loop, as will be explained in section 4.4.1.1.

For each joint, a specific controller used in WOTAS performs an internal control loop of the motor velocity. Two external loops close around this internal loop: one for feedback and controlling the interaction force between the exoskeleton and limb (lower loop); the other loop is responsible for applying forces to alter the upper-limb biomechanical parameters for suppressing the tremor (upper loop). The force value, τ_dd, which is introduced into the internal force loop, is calculated by adding the actions of the two external loops:

$$\tau_d = f_{dt} - f_{mt} + f_{dv} - \tau = f_{dt} - k_i q_t - k_v \dot{q}_t + f_d v - \tau \tag{4.1}$$

The upper part of the proposed control loop is responsible for altering the apparent impedance of the upper limb. It uses the information from the gyroscopes on the *Data treatment block* to distinguish between voluntary and tremor motion from the overall movement (as explained in the previous section). The angular velocity information from the estimated tremorous component is subsequently multiplied by the coefficients K_i and K_v, which define the apparent inertia and damping characteristics of each upper-limb joint. This process defines the actual impedance force of the system which is set to reduce the tremor. From these coefficients and the information filtered from each upper-limb joint movement (so that only information on the tremor is fed back) the force (f_{mt}) applied on the arm is calculated. This force tends to disappear as the tremor is suppressed. Thus, the difference between the calculated force, f_{mt}, and the desired force, f_{dt}, will tend to zero because in our application the f_{dt} value is selected as zero.

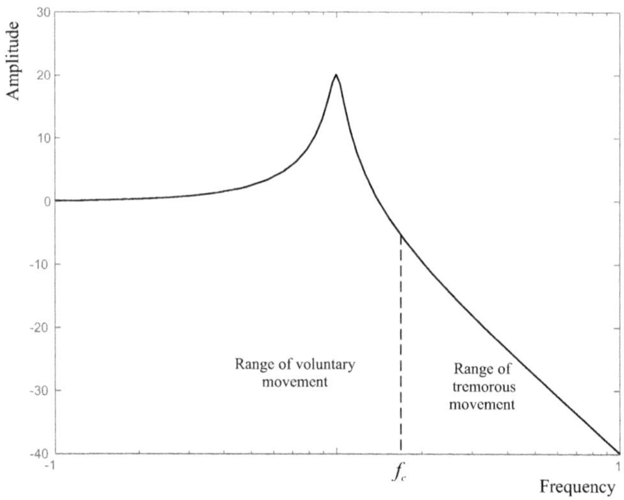

Fig. 4.10 The musculoskeletal system is modelled as a second-order biomechanical systems. The robotic exoskeleton is used to modify the apparent biomechanical characteristics of the upper limb so that the cutoff frequency, f_C, lies between the frequency ranges and tremor motion.

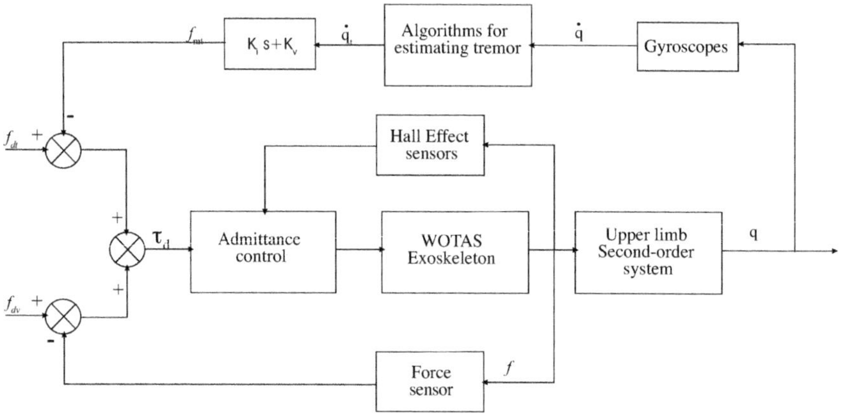

Fig. 4.11 Control strategy for altering upper-limb biomechanical parameters implemented in each WOTAS exoskeleton joint.

The lower loop of Figure 4.11 serves the goal of minimizing the effect of the exoskeleton on the voluntary motion. In this case, force sensors collect the interaction force between exoskeleton and the upper limb (τ). Under ideal circumstances, a user free of pathologic tremor should feel no force from the orthosis, i.e. no loading should be a consequence of voluntary motion. In order to achieve this, the interaction force, f, is filtered so that just force opposing voluntary motion is fed back in the lower branch of the control loop.

4.4.1.1 Force Control

In order to implement the control strategy for suppressing the tremor through impedance control a force controller was used in each of the WOTAS exoskeleton joints, i.e. each joint has a controller that is independent of the other upper-limb joints. We can thus consider our control system as a system in the joint space because the input reference values for each controller are in the joint and not the Cartesian space. This means that the control system proposed in this work differs from the majority of force control algorithms described in the literature. This is perhaps because nearly all the literature has been generated in the field of industrial manipulator robots and teleoperation, fields where robot tasks are defined in the Cartesian space.

One of the few works in which a force controller is studied in joint space dates back to the 1980s, [84], and it concludes that force controllers in the Cartesian space are preferable, because real-world tasks require divergent accommodations in the different Cartesian directions. Recently, [40], an impedance controller designed in the joint space has been presented. Another example of force control in the joint space is the one implemented in the exoskeleton developed by Culmer for the rehabilitation of patients with motor problems, [25]. The force measured by the sensors on the exoskeleton (task space) are converted into variables in the joint space for controlling each joint. Save these exceptions, nearly all authors place the force controller in the task space (Cartesian), specifying different control parameters for the different directions defined by the task. They thereby aim to obtain specific impedance in each direction of the task space. This is appropriate for many cases, but it must not be assumed that it is the best approach for all cases. In particular, joint control was chosen for the WOTAS exoskeleton, as will be explained below.

The joint control instead of Cartesian control approach is justified because it is a simpler approach and because individual control loops can be implemented in each joint with a high dynamic range, [132]. Moreover, the fact that each exoskeleton joint attempts to suppress the tremor generated at its level is interesting since it reduces the tremor in each joint. Thus, the problem of coupling the tremor between the different upper-limb joints is tackled. In chapter 2 of this book it was shown that in a large number of patients tremor movement displaces along the kinematic chain of the arm when its effects are reduced (by applying biomechanical loads) on one of the arm joints. However, the study of tremor behaviour when its effects are cancelled in different arm joints has still not been properly studied, [108]. Therefore, the factors affecting the functioning and stability of the force controller vary more from joint to joint than from Cartesian direction to Cartesian direction. This aspect led to devising active and independent control strategies in each joint. Thus, if cancelling the tremor in one of the joints increases the tremor in the other joint, the algorithm responsible for controlling the adjacent joint will identify the increased tremor (using the algorithms given in chapter 3) and will attempt to reduce the tremor generated by coupling the upper-limb joints. The aim then is that the active behaviour for reducing the tremor in each joint reaches equilibrium, thereby decreasing the coupling effects of the upper-limb joints.

Another important point in implementing the force controller of the WOTAS exoskeleton is the fact that the force sensor may be considered as a collocated sensor. A force sensor is said to be collocated when there is no distribution of masses and flexibilities between the actuator and sensor. In particular, when the only mass separating the actuator from the sensor is the rotor inertia, then the force sensor is collocated, [38]. This work considers that the WOTAS force sensors are directly collocated after joint elasticity, without any intermediary masses. In fact, joint elasticity is indistinguishable from environment elasticity, both are seen in a continuum, because as highlighted, virtually no mass of the links is seen from the actuator side. The force sensor is thus a collocated sensor that directly measures the elastic deformation produced by the actuator on joint transmission and the environment.

The fact that the force sensor is a collocated sensor has a number of advantages such as decreasing the negative effects of static friction and sensor noise on force control stability. Townsend and Salisbury, [131], determined that, in a force control loop, static friction and Coulombs friction may cause the exerted force to enter into a limit cycle. Another important issue is the effect of angular elasticity on force control. Pratt, [93], determines that elasticity partly transforms the force control problem into an actuator position/velocity control problem, as will be described in the following section of this chapter.

Admittance Control

The main objective of each joint controller is to control the interaction force between the exoskeleton and human body at each moment, thereby controlling the force applied by the actuators on the human body. The force and impedance controllers can be designed according to how the measured signals and control variables are used, i.e. the position, velocity and force magnitudes, and according to their relationship in the control diagram. This, in turn, depends on the application demands, the mechanical properties of the system and the electronic components used. The most common designs can be found in [117].

$$\dot{q} = f(F_{measured} - F_{desired}) \tag{4.2}$$

The WOTAS exoskeleton actuation system is implemented with flat brushless DC motors coupled to a harmonic drive as actuator elements. The controller executes an internal control loop to regulate the motor velocity from the information provided by the Hall effect sensors located in the motor structure. The velocity reference value, the control sign, is established via an external voltage, and from this reference value and the Hall sensor information, the controller generates a number of PWM pulses to control the motor velocity. Thus, in order to control the force applied by the actuator on the environment, an admittance control will adopt a controller from the group of force or impedance controllers using the position/velocity control, which indicates that the desired behaviour is implemented with external loops to control the force around an internal position or velocity loop. The force loop proposed in this work is therefore called admittance controller, [139], because from the force measurements, a velocity is set for the actuator, equation 4.2, [25]. The admittance controller was also used by Whitney, [139], for controlling damping, De Schutter and Van Brussel, [123], for pure force control (without any parallel position inputs), Klein et al. (1983) for an axis, or Gorinevsky and Schneider (1990) for force-impedance control on three axes. Although in the strict sense, the words *admittance* and *impedance* are antonyms, in a broad sense impedance control is everything that establishes a relationship between force, position and its derivatives. In this work the force applied by the exoskeleton on the upper limb is controlled via the motor velocity control, so that the impedance control of the limb-exoskeleton set is implemented using an admittance control strategy, [127].

One of the advantages of admittance controllers is that, unlike impedance controllers or controllers using torque control, they do not require a model of the system dynamics to be controlled. The main advantage of force control using torque control applied by the actuator is the speed in tracking the reference signal, [137]. However, these controllers are highly sensitive to friction and other uncertainties, [117]. Furthermore, admittance controllers enable the actuators to be used as velocity generators. Of course, this is only possible if the system conditions allow: high reductions and elasticities, [118].

In several earlier works, [84, 118], it has been shown that if the bandwidth of the internal velocity loop is much greater than the bandwidth of the external loop, the velocity/position-based schemes are more robust and less sensitive to disturbances than control methods using torque control. Moreover, if the position sensor is placed, as is usually done, next to the actuator output, thereby leaving all the structural flexibilities outside the control loop closed by the sensor, this internal loop admits very high control gains, [84]. Thus, this internal rigid position/velocity loop may reject non-modelled dynamic effects and disturbances of any other origin to a large extent, [123], including gravitational and friction effects, without explicitly compensating them. Therefore, the internal control loop provides the external control loop impedance with a system that has been filtered or cleaned and which is easy to control.

Most of the force control systems using position/velocity control proposed in the literature are designed to guarantee precision when a static force is applied by the system on the environment, [118]. In our case, the controller must be able to track dynamic force reference values because of the dynamic nature of the algorithms given in the previous section. Accordingly, the force control system proposed by Roy, [117], was adopted, which guarantees stable tracking of a dynamic force reference value, as long as the internal velocity controller is stable and able to track the velocity reference values generated within a bandwidth. In this work three distinct controllers are proposed and their tracking of dynamic force reference values is evaluated. Finally, the stability of each of the proposed controllers is analysed and evaluated. As a result, Roy defends that the best controller is the feedforward admittance controller from the force profile of the controller input.

Another aspect to be considered is the effects of the oscillations and characteristics of the control system on force controller response when the robot is in contact with the environment. It is known that when a robot comes into contact with the environment, the interaction forces not only depend on the velocity of the impact, but also on the impedance (rigidity and inertia) of the impact, [54, 90]. Therefore, the greater the impedance of the mechanism, the greater the interaction forces will be for small disturbances. In our system, the exoskeleton is always in contact with the environment (human upper limb), i.e. there is always a contact force, f, between the exoskeleton and limb. Moreover, the contact environment (human upper arm) has an elasticity (soft human tissues) that reduces the negative effects of the force controllers, [79]. Furthermore, this contact elasticity reduces the bandwidth of the controlled system, [55, 120]. When the exoskeleton is in contact with the environment the following hypotheses can be formulated, [57]:

1. The effect of the contact force on the internal velocity control loop is negligible due to the fact that the reducer used is not backdrivable. Thus, the velocity tracking error converges asymptotically to zero.
2. The environment is sufficiently elastic (soft tissues) so that the contact force acts as a disturbance limited to the system. This leads to a velocity tracking error of limited range.

Thus, the task is to design an external force control loop that generates velocity reference values, within a bandwidth, for the internal velocity control loop. Therefore, the system will be able to track dynamic force reference values asymptotically and exactly, [68]. The control algorithm developed for WOTAS is the one depicted in figure 4.12.

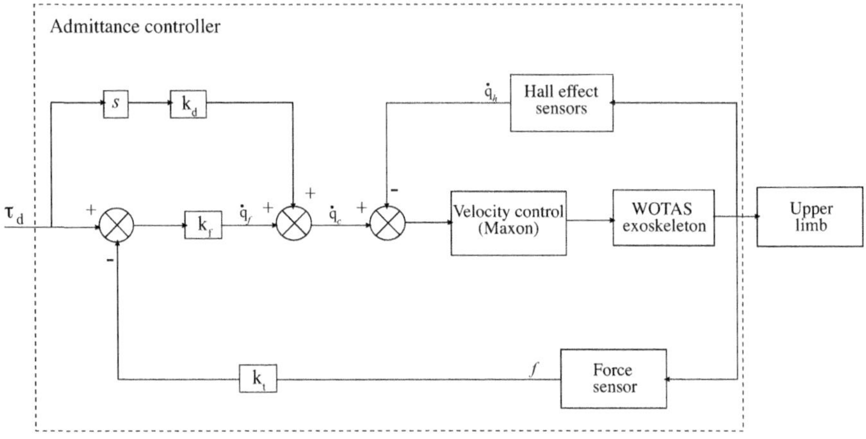

Fig. 4.12 Admittance controller implemented in the WOTAS exoskeleton

In accordance with this algorithm, the velocity reference value velocity, q_c, which is introduced into the internal velocity control loop is calculated using the following control law, [118]:

$$\dot{q}_c = k_d \dot{\tau}_d - k_f \Delta\tau = k_d \dot{\tau}_d - k_f(\tau_d - \tau) \quad (4.3)$$

In this equation, $\Delta\tau$ is the interaction force error in each joint. τ_d is the dynamic torque reference value, i.e. the torque value that is to be applied on the arm. τ is the torque value applied by the exoskeleton on the arm. This value is obtained by multiplying the value measured by the force sensor, f, which measures the interaction force between the exoskeleton and the upper limb, by a factor k_t that transforms the value measured in volts into a physical value in $N.m$. Both τ and τ_d are expressed in joint values. k_f is the proportional gain of the force controller and k_d the force control feedforward loop gain. The internal velocity control loop uses the information from the Hall sensors coupled to the motor axis, $\dot{q}_h$.

The controller proposed in 4.3 guarantees stable tracking asymptotically of a dynamic force reference value as long as the internal velocity control loop is stable and able to track the velocity reference values generated by the external force control loop, [117, 118]. This condition is satisfied by the velocity controller used in WOTAS.

The controller proposed has a feedforward control loop to control the force applied by the robotic device on the limb. The function of this loop is to minimise the tracking errors of a dynamic force reference value when feedforwarding the internal velocity control loop with an estimate of the desired velocity, [118]. The advantages of the feedforward control loop will be explained in the next section during the evaluation and selection of the parameters of the proposed control algorithm. The action of the feedforward controller loop is combined with the advantages of the feedback control loop, responsible for correcting the error measured between the applied and measured force, 4.2. Thus it can be said that the force control algorithm of the WOTAS robot is a controller with two degrees of freedom, [68]. The parameters of the proposed control system were experimentally adjusted with very good results as shown in the next section.

4.4.1.2 Experimental Results

This section describes three experiments that illustrate the behaviour and selection of the parameters of the admittance controller proposed in the previous section. The results presented in this section were obtained during the adjustment tests of the actuator controller responsible for activating the WOTAS exoskeleton elbow joint. The architecture for programming the control strategies, sensors and actuators are those given in section 4.3. The WOTAS elbow joint was adjusted to a user to evaluate the proposed controller, figure 4.8.

The functioning of the controller-actuator system can be evaluated using different functioning metrics, e.g. maximum force, force resolution, position resolution, actuator inertia, force precision (controllable force), force bandwidth, position bandwidth and force distortion, [90]. It is important to choose the appropriate metrics for each application, i.e. those that evaluate the relevant aspects of the task to be done by the operator. In the case of the WOTAS exoskeleton for cancelling tremor, it is interesting to quantify the range of controllable forces and system response in tracking reference values.

In order to evaluate the functioning of the proposed system, itwo experiments have been defined in which the aforementioned characteristics are evaluated. The experiments, results and conclusions of the evaluation of the controlled system metrics will be described in the following sections.

Evaluation of Tracking Dynamic Force Reference Values

To evaluate the system behaviour in tracking force profiles, different dynamic force reference values were programmed in the WOTAS admittance controller which obey the following equation:

$$\tau_d = A\sin(2\pi ft) \tag{4.4}$$

In an earlier study by the author in tremor patients it was shown that the torque of tremor movements in each joint usually occurs in a frequency range of up to 8 Hz, [112]. Accordingly, different algorithms were programmed for tracking reference values at different frequencies. In this same study the mean torque values for tremor movement in each joint were evaluated. It was thus defined that the force reference value to be followed had an amplitude, A, of 1 $N.m$.

In this section the action of the feedforward control loop will be evaluated. For this, the results of the two controllers will be compared, one without the feedforward control loop (CP) and another with the feedforward control loop (CPF). The results are shown in figure 4.13. In this figure each controller response and reference value can be seen. Moreover, the tracking error of each controller force profile is shown. It can also be observed how algorithm response considerably differs, primarily as the frequency of the reference signal increases. For force profiles of up to 1 Hz it can be seen in the figure that both controllers have an excellent response with an almost negligible phase error, about 2 degrees and an amplitude error always lower then 1,5%. For force profiles of up to 3 Hz the force tracking error is not so large for the two controllers evaluated, although it can be observed that the controller with anticipative action has a better response. In the case of the CP controller, the error was approximately $\pm 10\%$, whereas for the CPF controller, the error was not greater than $\pm 2.5\%$.

However, on increasing the reference signal frequency to 6 Hz (figure 4.13c) both controllers perform worse, especially the controller CP. At this frequency, the CP controller amplitude error is $\pm 20\%$ and the CPF, $\pm 5\%$. For force reference values with 9 Hz frequency the error increases further, reaching $\pm 55\%$ for the CP controller and $\pm 20\%$ for the CPF controller.

These results show that the admittance controller feedforward loop functions considerably better, enabling dynamic force reference values of up to 6-8 Hz with a relatively low error to be applied. It is known that the majority of tremor movements usually occur in a range of 3-8 Hz, [108]. Accordingly, the controller designed and

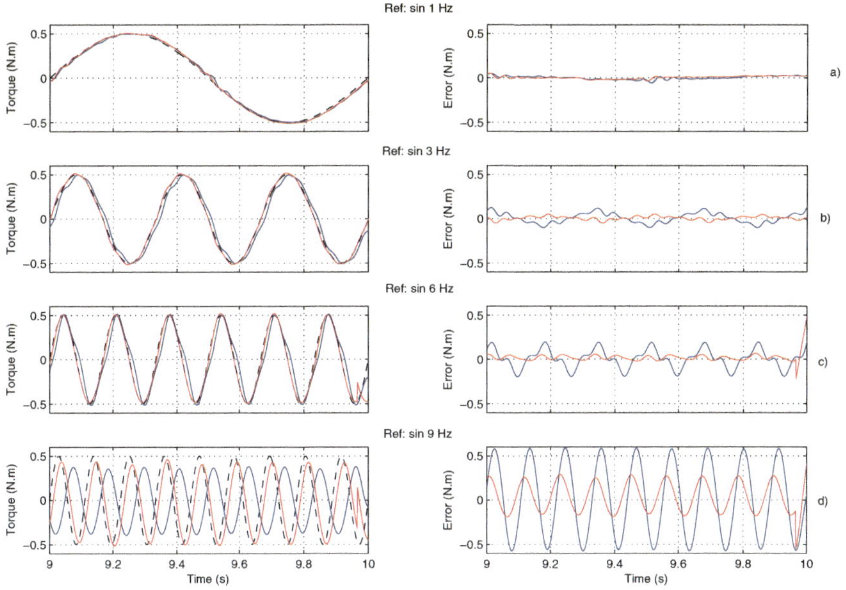

Fig. 4.13 Response of the two force controllers evaluated, CF (blue) and CPF (red), and dynamic force profiles at different frequencies. Left: force reference values and controller response; Right: force profile tracking errors

presented in this section has the right speed response and precision to be used in a robotic exoskeleton for suppressing tremor.

Evaluation of the Tracking of Human Voluntary Arm Joint Movements

The functioning of the robot force controller in tracking voluntary movements of the upper-limb joints has also been evaluated in this work. For this, WOTAS was adapted to different users and the parameters f_{dt} and f_{dv} (figure 4.11) were adjusted to zero, so that the controllers prevented the exoskeleton from applying forces on the upper limb at any moment. Thus, the force measured by the sensors must be as close to zero as possible.

As a protocol for evaluating the experiments a number of tasks were defined for the user, and the interaction force between the exoskeleton and limb at each instant was measured. The tasks selected were: with the arm at rest, touching the end of the nose with the index finger, touching objects and drawing a spiral. Thus algorithm response for different tasks at different execution frequencies was tested. Figure 4.14 depicts the system response. In this figure it can be observed that the torque that the exoskeleton applies on the arm is never greater than 80 $mN.m$. This is an acceptable result because this value is barely noticeable for human touch. Moreover, as will see in the next chapter, the subjective rating of the different WOTAS users indicates that reaction forces were not felt from the exoskeleton on their natural movement.

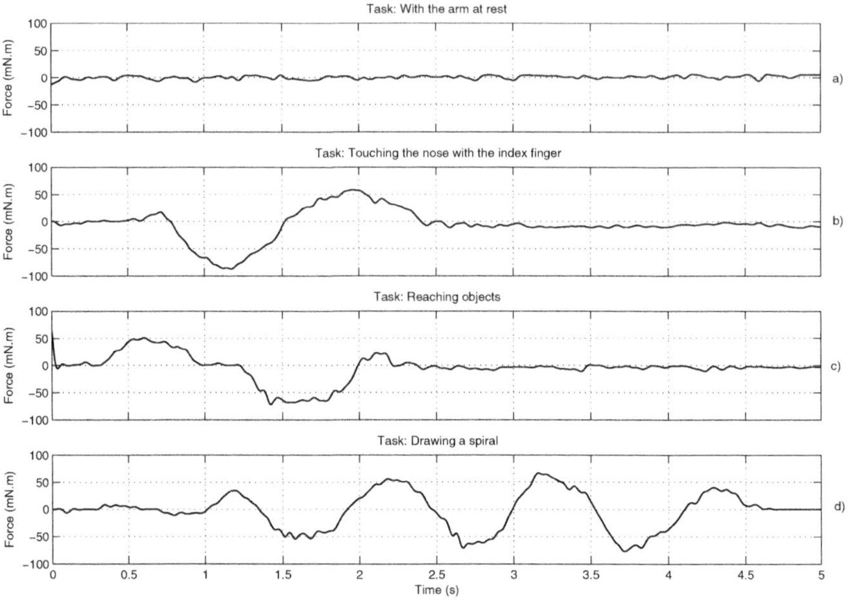

Fig. 4.14 Algorithm response in free functioning mode.

Furthermore, the system was also evaluated in a user doing daily office tasks. This user used the exoskeleton, also with the parameters f_{dt} and f_{dv} adjusted to zero, for several minutes doing daily tasks in the usual way. After this period, the user said that he did not notice the application of forces on his voluntary movements. A part of this period of time is depicted in figure 4.15. As can be observed in the figure, at no moment was the torque applied by the exoskeleton on the arm greater than 70 $mN.m$.

4.4.2 Exploitation of the Repetitive Characteristics of Tremor Movement

Tremor is usually described in the bibliography as a rhythmical and involuntary contraction characterised by oscillations at a central frequency, [7]. Tremor frequency varies according to the particular neurological disorder being considered. In particular, while essential tremor takes place in the frequency range between 5 and 8 Hz, rest tremor is usually found at a slightly lower frequency range, 3 to 6 Hz.

Moreover, for a given type of tremor, its main frequency varies from patient to patient, but tends to be quite stable for a particular subject. This property should be exploited when designing a control strategy to counteract tremor. In particular, repetitive control (RC) can handle periodic (repetitive) signals and disturbances, [8]. Repetitive control can be regarded as a subset of learning control since the control action is determined using the stored error values from preceding periods.

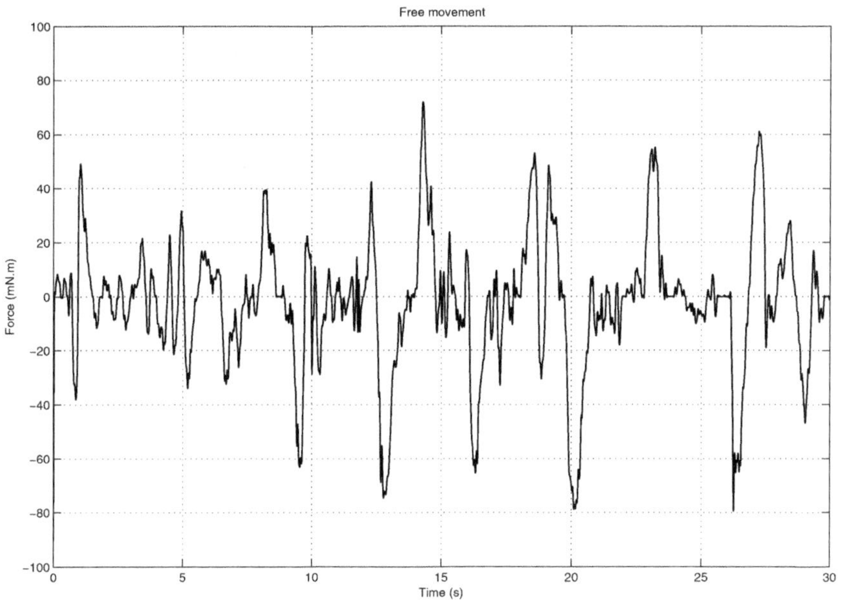

Fig. 4.15 Algorithm interaction torque response in free functioning mode with the patient moving at random.

Even though repetitive approaches can handle periodic signals (tremor), it is not free from some common problems: tight stability conditions, poor response to non-periodic and non-harmonic signals and poor noise characteristics. As reported by Inoue, [63], a stabilizing compensation and smoothing of the control signal over periods can be used to overcome the above mentioned problems.

In this kind of control systems a function approximator " is used whereby input and output correspondence is adapted during control, so that a desired behaviour of the system is obtained, [136]. In the case of repetitive control, the function approximator consists of a memory loop that learns the signal behaviour whenever it is periodical. In order to further understand the behaviour of the system, figure 4.16 shows the Bode diagram of the typical repetitive controller. As can be observed in the figure, repetitive control implements a notch filter (infinite attenuation) on the input signal at frequency ω_0. This, of course, is the behaviour to be achieved, i.e. to have a maximum attenuation at the disturbance frequency. However, this is obtained at the expense of a poor attenuation (even gain) at intermediate frequencies. Another consequence of the sharp attenuation peaks is the susceptibility of the system to stability problems, [63].

The idea behind this approach is that the control strategy manage the exoskeleton to generate a motion equal but opposite to the tremor, based on the real time estimation of the involuntary component of motion described in chapter 3, actively compensating and effectively subtracting the tremor for the overall motion.

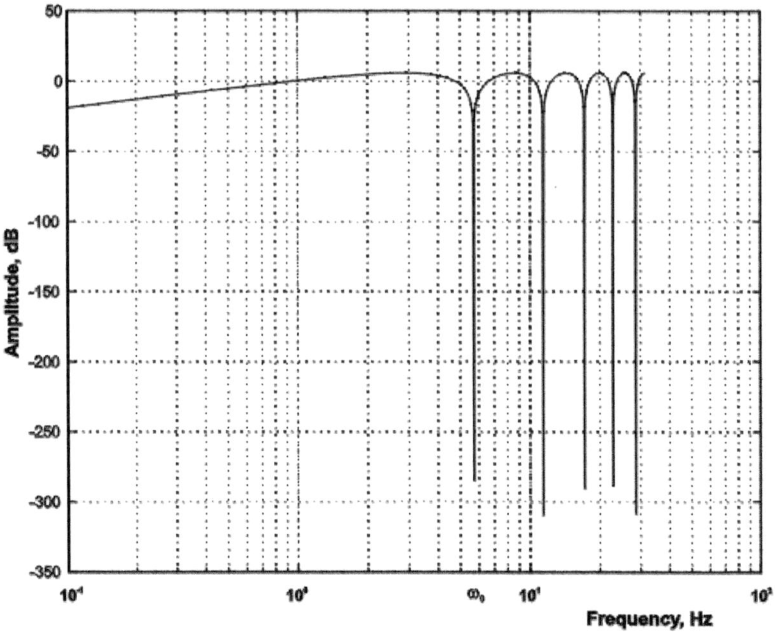

Fig. 4.16 An active notch lter is implemented by means of the active orthosis. In this scheme the notch lter frequency, ω, lies exactly at the tremor frequency.

4.4.2.1 Implementation of a Notch Filter at Tremor Movement Frequency

In order to implement the active controller from the repetitive control for suppressing the tremor an approximation of joint control is also used, i.e. each joint is controlled independently to minimise the coupling problems of the tremor in the different upper-limb joints. The control strategy designed and proposed in this book for active control of the pathological tremor is depicted in figure 4.17. In the control strategy proposed the velocity of each human upper-limb joint is controlled, [140]. The velocity reference value velocity, q_c, which is introduced into the velocity control loop, is calculated using the following control law:

$$\dot{q_c} = \dot{q_f} + \dot{q_{tr}} = k_f(f_{dv} - f) + (\dot{q_{dt}} + z^{-M_k} \cdot \dot{q}_t) \tag{4.5}$$

As in the passive approach, this strategy also consists of a dual control loop. The upper loop is responsible for actively suppressing the tremor, whereas the lower loop is responsible for reducing the effects of biomechanical load on natural movement, [113].

In the upper loop, the algorithm given in chapter 3 estimates the velocity of the tremor movement, $\dot{q}_t$. The amplitude of the velocity of the tremor movement has a delay of M seconds. M is defined by equation 4.6, where ω_s is the sample frequency of the control strategy and ω_t is the estimated tremor frequency. Thus, the amplitude of the tremor movement, added to a velocity reference value, $\dot{q_{dt}}$, is fed

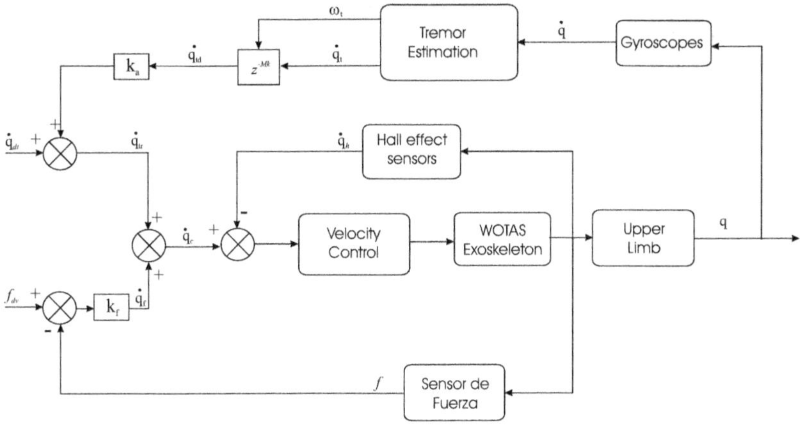

Fig. 4.17 Active tremor suppression control strategy: Velocity repetitive control strategy implemented in the WOTAS exoskeleton.

back to the WOTAS exoskeleton internal velocity controller. The WOTAS actuators will therefore describe a velocity profile of equal amplitude but in counter phase to the estimated tremor movement, actively cancelling and effectively subtracting the tremor from the total movement of the user. For this, in our system, the velocity reference value, $\dot{q}_{dt}$, is adjusted to zero. The value of the constant k_a defines the amplitude of the movement that will be fed back to the velocity controller.

$$M = \omega_s / \omega_t \tag{4.6}$$

The lower loop is in charge of reducing the application of loads on voluntary movement. For this, an admittance control is implemented, i.e. the sensors measure the interaction force between the exoskeleton and upper limb, f, which multiplied by the force control loop gain, k_f , defines the velocity reference value $\dot{q}_f$ that is fed back to the WOTAS internal motor velocity controller. As already mentioned, in ideal conditions, a patient without tremors must not note any resistance to natural arm movement from the robotic device. For this, as in the case of passive control proposed in the previous section, the reference value that defines the force applied on the voluntary movement of the user, f_{dv}, is adjusted to zero. As in the previous control approach, the quality of the tremor suppression control approach is strongly dependent on accurate estimation and tracking of tremor frequency. In [113] it is shown that the system is stable when the algorithm for tremor estimation is stable.

As explained in the previous paragraph, unlike the passive approach, in which the energy of the tremor movement is dissipated, in the active approach energy is transferred (in counter phase to the tremor movement) to the system. In accordance with the bibliographical review in this book, [108], the active approach of suppressing tremor has never been implemented in any system for this purpose. The system proposed is new and its effectiveness in suppressing the pathological tremor and its effects on users will be evaluated in this book in trials with patients. The system has an adaptive behaviour so that constantly (in real time) it updates both the estimate of the tremor amplitude and its frequency. The system is thus capable of responding to changes produced by the control strategy on the tremor. Moreover, as it controls each joint independently, it manages to uncouple the tremor from the different upper-limb joints.

4.4.2.2 Experimental Results

This section describes the experiments that illustrate the behaviour and selection of the parameters of the controller proposed in the previous section. The results presented in this section were obtained during the adjustment tests of the actuator controller responsible for activating the WOTAS exoskeleton elbow joint. The architecture for programming the control strategies, sensors and actuators are those given in section 4.3.

As seen in section 4.2.3, the maximum torque value applied by the DC-reducer motor set was adjusted to 3 $N.m$ (the estimated torque value associated with tremor movement, [112]). The system is thus prevented from applying more force than is necessary for suppressing the tremor, thereby guaranteeing the safety of the exoskeleton user. However, for the tests proposed in this section, the maximum value of the torque applied on the upper limb was altered. This is because, during the tests, the actuator system will have to move the entire arm at very high frequencies. It is known that the musculoskeletal system of the human upper limb functions as a low-pass filter, [59, 92]. In order to overcome the effect of this filter and make the arm move at higher frequencies the torque value applied by the actuator system was adjusted to its maximum value of 8 $N.m$. Likewise, for the tests the user was asked to have his arm has free as possible, i.e. not applying any voluntary forces counter to the movement imposed by the exoskeleton.

The metrics used for evaluating the functioning of the controller proposed in this section was that with the system the elbow joint achieved velocity reference values at frequencies within the range of the tremor frequencies. In our application it is interesting to quantify the range of controllable velocities and system velocity response to tracking reference values. The experiments and results of the evaluation of the controlled system metrics will be described in the following section.

Evaluation of the System Tracking of Dynamic Velocity Reference Values

In order to suppress the tremor with a notch filter the system actuators must move in counter phase to the tremor movement estimated in each joint. In earlier studies the author detected that tremor movements occur in a frequency range between 3-8 Hz at a maximum angular velocity of roughly 2.5 rad/s, [112]. Therefore, to evaluate system behaviour in velocity profile tracking, different dynamic velocity reference values were programmed in the WOTAS velocity controller with the following form:

$$\tau_d = A\sin(2\pi f t) \tag{4.7}$$

The experimentation conditions are the same as those above. Thus algorithm tracking of the velocity profiles at different frequencies was evaluated. The results obtained are shown in figure 4.18.

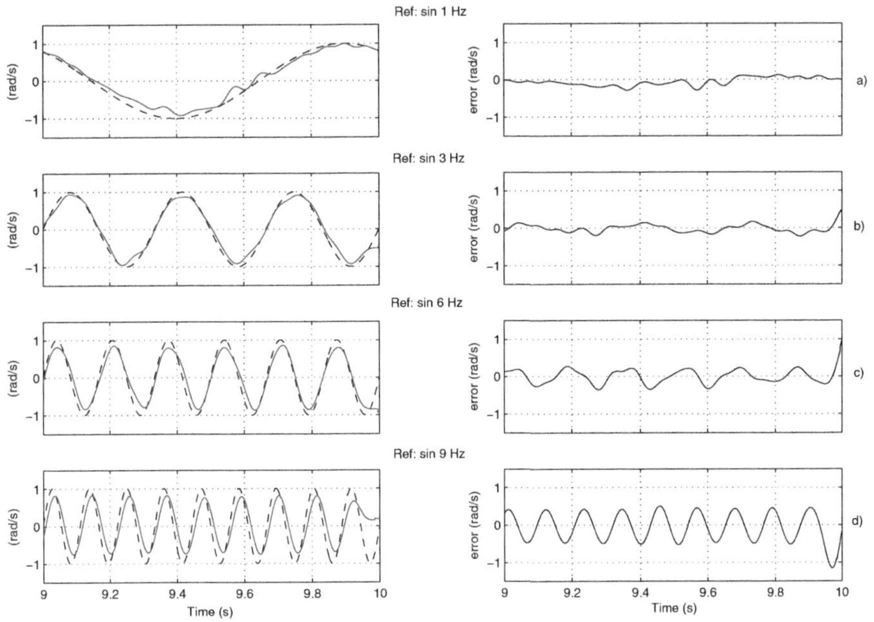

Fig. 4.18 Velocity control response implemented in the WOTAS exoskeleton with a dynamic velocity reference value at different frequencies: a) 1 Hz b) 3 Hz c) 6 Hz d) 9 Hz. Left: velocity reference signals (black) and system response (blue). Right: velocity profile tracking errors.

In figure 4.18 it can be observed that the system is able to track dynamic velocity reference values up to movements of 6 Hz. In other words, the system is capable of inducing movements of up to 6 Hz on each active joint of the exoskeleton. For the frequency of 6 Hz, error between the movement induced on the arm and the reference is 15 %. This value is acceptable given how complicated it is to apply dynamic forces on soft body tissues, [85]. However, on increasing the frequency of the reference value to 9 Hz, figure 4.18d, the error between the arm movement and the velocity reference value increases, reaching $\pm 30\%$. This high value is due to the filter of high frequency movements in the human musculoskeletal system, [92].

The torque mean values for generating movement to cancel the tremor in each joint were evaluated in this same study. The torque value in each joint, τ, is defined as, [71]:

$$\tau = J \cdot \alpha \tag{4.8}$$

where J is the moment of inertia of the arm segment connected to the joint and α is the value of angular acceleration of the joint movement. Thus, the required torque value for generating movements in human joints increases in proportion to the

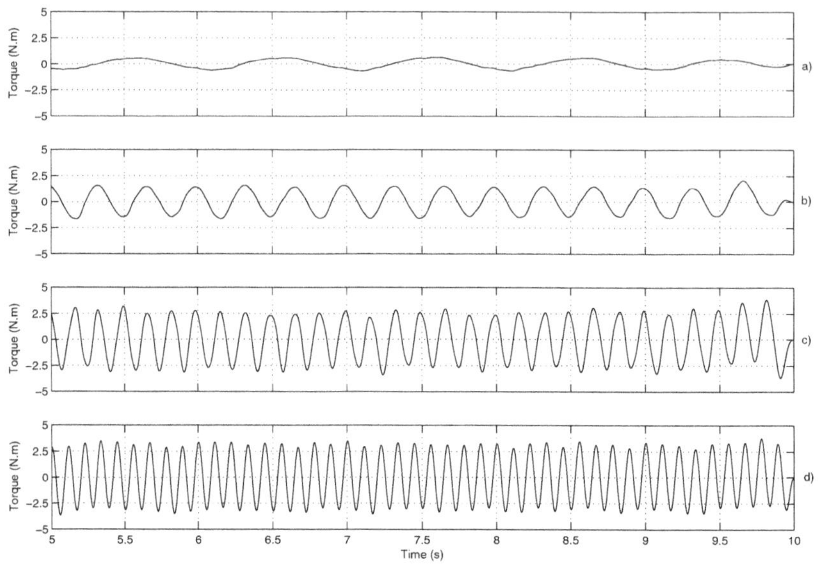

Fig. 4.19 Torque values applied by the WOTAS exoskeleton to generate movements on the elbow joint of a patient. The increased torque value required to track the reference values at high frequencies is considerable.

increase in frequency. This behaviour is depicted in figure 4.19 where the increased torque value required by the actuator system to generate movements at greater frequencies can be observed. These values vary from patient to patient since they are related to the moment of inertia of the arm segment, J, and this value is defined by the anthropometrical characteristics of each individual, [112].

In figure 4.19 it can also be observed that the system presents a maximum value of movement transmission the arm joint. The torque values required for tracking reference values at frequencies of 6 Hz and 9 Hz are very similar. This is because the soft tissues, for these high frequencies, filter nearly all movement produced by the exoskeleton, i.e. although the exoskeleton is generating high-frequency movements (9 Hz), not all this movement is transmitted to the human skeleton, as the movements generated by the robotic exoskeleton are absorbed by the skin surface movements, [12].

The behaviour of the lower loop for tracking the voluntary movements of the patient was evaluated in the section above, where it was shown that the exoskeleton is able to work in free mode without affecting the natural movements of the user, by applying a barely noticeable resistance of 80 $N.m$.

4.5 Conclusions

This chapter presented a robotic exoskeleton able to monitor, diagnose and control tremor in subjects. This robotic exoskeleton is equipped with kinematic and kinetic sensors for the measurement and calculation of joint angular displacement, velocity and acceleration, as well as interaction forces between the limb and orthosis. In addition, it could also apply dynamic force to the articulations of the upper limb by means of a set of flat dc motors in combination with pancake gears. The big innovations of the WOTAS exoskeleton are its portability, its non invasiveness, and that it provides direct information from each joint of the upper limb.

In order to achieve the objectives defined for this chapter, two control strategies were designed and implemented for suppressing tremor movements with robotic exoskeletons. A passive control strategy has been presented, which absorbs tremor movement energy by altering the impedance of the musculoskeletal system and applying dissipating forces to the tremor. The other control strategy proposed is based on a new approach for suppressing tremor: adding energy to the system in counter phase to the tremor. The second approach has never been used for cancelling tremor and its efficiency in real patients will be presented in the next chapter. The controllability range of both control strategies proposed was evaluated in this chapter and they have shown to be able to generate the forces required for suppressing tremor.

In summary, the operation of WOTAS system for tremor suppression is based on the identification of tremorous motion out of the kinematics and kinetics sensor reading. Adaptive algorithms help identify and distinguish tremorous motion from the voluntary one. This information is then used to establish a proper physical interaction (modification of the combined human-exoskeleton articular impedance or applying forces opposite to tremor) that should result in tremor reduction.

The main contribution of the chapter has been the design of new control strategies. These differ from the control strategies found in the literature where the cancelling action of the tremor does not affect the voluntary movements of the exoskeleton user. Moreover, the adaptive behaviour of the control strategies proposed mean that the tremor is suppressed at the same level where it is evident: in joints. This means that there exist no coordination between control loops at different joints. As a result of this, tremor migration is immediately detected and tracked at any of the proximal joints. The consequence of this detection and tracking of tremor is the corresponding counteraction. The mutual adaptation process was used to decouple the influence of tremor at adjacent joints, which results in an overall reduction of proximally migrated tremor, [113]. In addition, the range of movement of each articulation of the exoskeleton is limited by the control strategies in such a way that they never exceeds the natural range of motion of the user. This was implemented in order to guarantee user safety. Moreover, the strategies proposed were designed for ambulatory devices, so they do not require any external reference point for suppressing the tremor.

In the next chapter the WOTAS exoskeleton and the control strategies presented in this chapter will be evaluated with patients suffering from tremor. The system proposed and the control strategies will help understand the mechanisms of tremor.

The capacity of applying internal dynamic forces to the upper limb opens widely the application field of WOTAS exoskeleton. It could be applied in different areas of the rehabilitation robotic field, for instance, it could provide restoration or maintenance of motor function to different joints of the upper limb. Most of the powered orthoses designed to date are nonambulatory devices, [65, 95]. There is a need in the rehabilitation area of ambulatory devices able to apply dynamic forces to the upper limb.

Chapter 5
Upper Limb Exoskeleton for Tremor Suppression: Validation

This chapter introduces the protocol for the validatation of the exoskeleton and control strategies introduced in previous chapters. This protocol is a set of tasks defined according the clinical criterias. In order to evaluate the performance of the device developed to suppress tremor we conducted an experimental phase involving 10 patients suffering from different tremor diseases. The clinical effectiveness and the user's acceptance was the criterias selected for the elaboration of the evaluation protocol.

5.1 Experimental Protocol

In order to evaluate the performance of the device developed to suppress tremor we conducted an experimental phase involving 10 patients suffering from different tremor diseases. The objectives of these experiments were to:

- Evaluate WOTAS exoskeleton
- Validate the developed tremor suppression control strategies
- Compare active and passive control strategies
- Determine the better combination of parameters for each joint

These experiments were conducted in Hôpital Erasme, in Belgium, and Hospital General Universitário de Valencia, in Spain, and were led by a neurologist. The protocol, the results and the analysis of the results are presented in the following sections.

5.1.1 Users

Ten users participated in these experiments (3 women, mean age 52,3 years). Users presented different pathologies but the majority was affected by Essential Tremor (ET). ET was moderate in users 1, 3, 4 and 7 and severe in users 2, 5, and 6. User 8 suffer from multiple sclerosis, user 9 from post-traumatic tremor and user 10 is

E. Rocon and J.L. Pons: Exoskeletons in Rehabilitation Robotics, STAR 69, pp. 99–111.
springerlink.com

affected by a mixed tremor. All users provided their informed consent. The investigation was approved by the ethical committee of both hospitals. All the experiments were recorded.

The users still exhibited tremor despite a regular intake of the drugs conventionally administered for tremor, even at high doses for some of the users.

5.1.2 Materials and Methods

Three different people were present during the measurements, see figure 5.1:

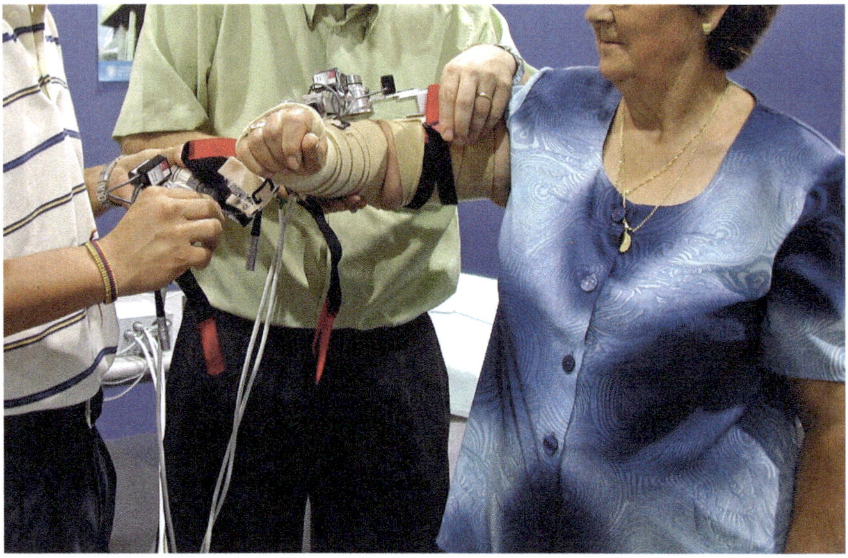

Fig. 5.1 Illustration of the process of placing WOTAS over the arm of a patient during experiments.

- *A computer operator:* In charge of setting the parameters of the systems and recording the signals.
- *A medical doctor:* In charge of supervision of the condition of the trials and the state of the user.
- *An experimenter:* In charge of fitting and removing the orthosis and interacting with the user to perform the trials.

The exoskeleton was evaluated in several sessions and it was adapted to the particularities of each user, as illustrated in figure 5.2.

During the experiments neither the user, nor the experimenter or the medical doctor knew when the systems were applying a suppressing strategy or when it was operating in monitoring mode. Just the computer operator knew when the systems were applying the suppression strategy. For formal purposes, we consider this

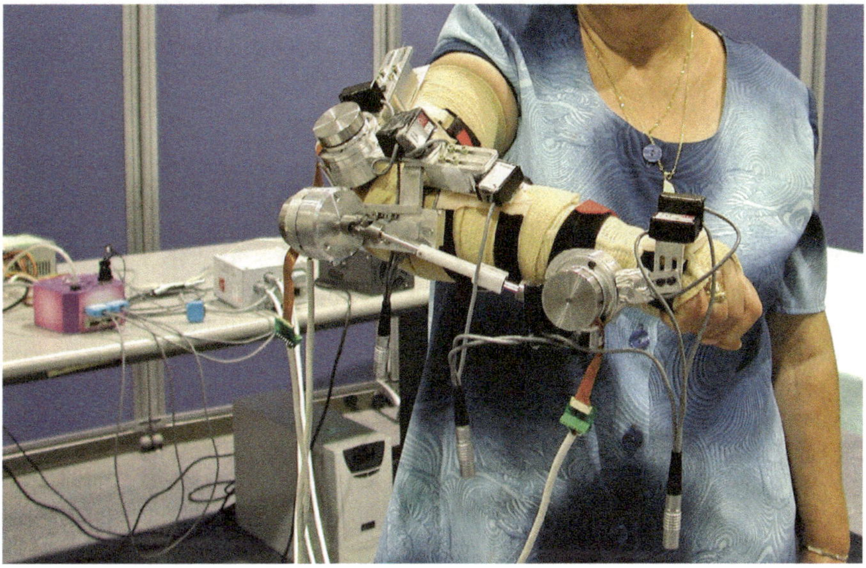

Fig. 5.2 Wotas placed over the arm of a patient.

arrangement equivalent to a double-blind trial in order to reduce the placebo effects in the experimentation phase, [13].

All the experiments were recorded for future analysis.

5.1.3 Tasks

Three different tasks were selected to be performed by the users: Keep the arm outstretched, point the nose with a finger, and keep the arm in a rest position. These tasks have been previously used to characterise tremor movement, [13].

During the experiments, WOTAS operated basically in its three different control modes as follows:

1. *Monitoring mode.* WOTAS operate in free mode (no force is applied on the upper limb) and monitor tremor parameters of the users.
2. *Passive Control mode.* WOTAS is able to change biomechanical characteristics of upper limb, such as viscosity or inertia, in order to suppress tremor (section 4.4.1).
3. *Active Control mode.* WOTAS is able to apply opposite forces to the tremorous movement based on a real time estimation of the involuntary component of motion (section 4.4.2).

The order in which the modes have been applied has been alternated, as well as the order in which the users have executed the tasks. In each experimental session, 3 repetitions of each task were realized. This approach was adopted in order to avoid interactions in the analysis, as well as learning effects, [13]. The number of repetitions has been chosen in order to have an experimental session not longer than 1 hour.

5.1.4 Data Analysis

The data analyzed were the output voltage coming from the gyroscopes placed on the active orthosis. This output voltage was sampled at a 2000 Hz rate. The data has been filtered using a Kernel Smoothing algorithm and a gaussian window 51 points width. The figure of merit adopted to quantify the reduction achieved by the exoskeleton is the ratio between the signal analyzed in monitoring mode (P_{mm}), and the signal analyzed in suppression mode (P_{sm}), both in passive or active modes, equation 5.1. Therefore, the reduction of tremor was measured with the users under the same conditions: with the orthosis placed on the upper limb. As a result, the estimated reduction was the remaining tremor in suppression mode referred to tremor at monitoring mode.

$$R = \frac{P_{sm}}{P_{mm}} \cdot 100 \tag{5.1}$$

The parameter selected to compare the tremor level is the Power contained in the frequency band from 2 Hz to 8 Hz, [108]. It can be defined as follows:

$$\Phi(f) = \frac{FFT(x)FFT(x)^*}{N} \tag{5.2}$$

$$P = \sum_{i=f_1}^{f_2} \frac{\Phi(i)}{T} = \frac{1}{Nt_s} \sum_{i=f_1}^{f_2} \Phi(i) \tag{5.3}$$

where x is the signal in the time domain, N is the length of the signal, t_s is the sampling period and, f_1 and f_2 are the lower and upper limits of the range of interest.

5.2 Results and Discussion

The effects of adding effective viscosity were investigated for the upper limb during the execution of the different tasks. During the trials, some users were able to identify when the system was operating in *suppression* mode, relating to the clinician either '*now the system is suppressing my tremor*' or '*now it is not*'.

Figure 5.3 illustrates the performance of WOTAS when operating in suppression mode for all subjects in this experiment. Notice that the efficiency of the exoskeleton improves with tremor power increase. An statistical analysis has been made to characterized the tremor suppression. The statistical analysis has been made using R, [99]. A second order polynomial fit has been made with the natural logarithms of power spectra in free and suppression mode, see red line on figure 5.4. As showed in table 5.1, the adjusted R^2 of the fitting is 0.44 and all the coefficients of the fitting are statistically significant at 0.05.

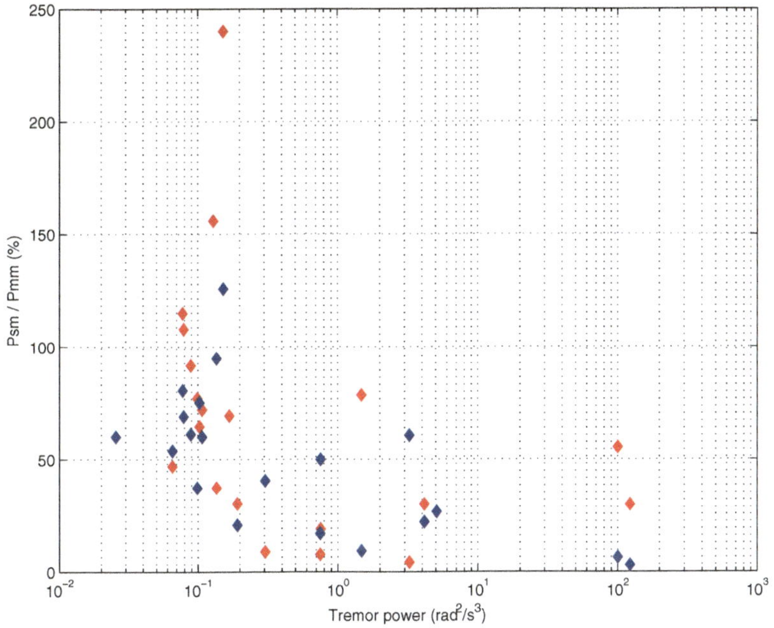

Fig. 5.3 Tremor reduction (*y axis*) achieved by WOTAS operating in suppressing both in active (blue markers) and passive (red markers), mode. *x axis* represents users' tremor energy with WOTAS in *monitoring* mode

Table 5.1 users information

	Estimate	Std. Error	t value	$P_r(>\mid t \mid)$
Intercept	-1.40	0.36	-3.87	0.0003
X	0.45	0.11	4.21	0.00012
X^2	0.09	0.04	2.34	0.024

From this fitting it is possible to estimate where the orthosis suppress tremor efficiently, based on finding the points where the fitting crosses the line y=x (green line on figure 5.4). This method allows us to identify a lower limit for efficient tremor suppression, this limit is roughly 0.15 $\frac{rad^2}{s^3}$. In Figure 5.3 we can check that the robotic exoskeleton has a minimum tremor suppression limit, i.e., if the spectral density of tremor movement is below the lower limit identified, around 0.15 $\frac{rad^2}{s^3}$, WOTAS exoskeleton is ineffective in suppressing the tremor.

In order to verify the hypothesis that over the lower limit (0.15 $\frac{rad^2}{s^3}$) WOTAS is efficient in tremor suppression, an univariate ANOVA analysis was performed.

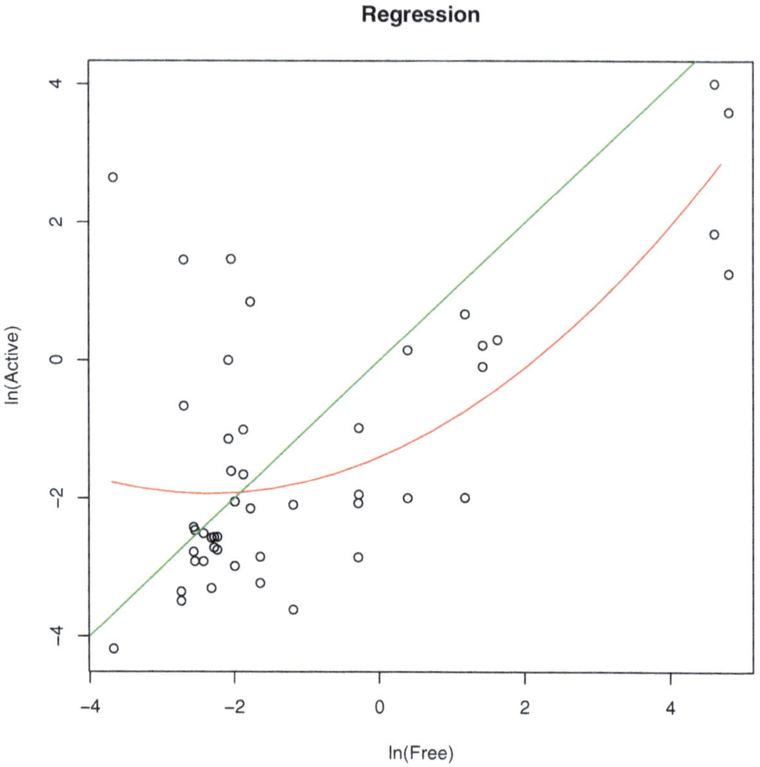

Fig. 5.4 Polynomial fitting to the data

This analysis was made for all movements which tremor in free mode was above the threshold obtained by the regression curve. The hypothesis is that the orthoses is efficient for severe cases of tremor, when tremor is small (under the threshold of 0.15 $\frac{rad^2}{s^3}$) the system has a negligible contribution. Five from the six users had movements in which the PSD of tremor was above the threshold and these are the measurements included in the analysis. The analysis was based on two factors: system in monitoring mode and system in suppression mode. Users were included to the model and the dependent variable was the Neperian Logarithm of the Power Spectral Density - Ln(PSD. The results of this ANOVA analysis are shown in table 5.2. According to the table, the effects due to the mode (active vs monitoring) as well as due to the user are statistically significant. Moreover, as we can see in figure 5.5, the active mode reduces the mean value of the Ln(PSD).

The user also have a significant effect on the Ln(PSD) but not on the interaction mode-user as showed in table 5.2. However, WOTAS demonstrated its effect in reducing the tremor component in all users with tremor superior to the threshold (figure 5.6)

Table 5.2 Results of the ANOVA analysis

Source		Type III Sum of squares	df	Mean Square	F	Sig.
Intercept	Hypothesis	11.42	1.00	11.42	0.42	0.56
	Error	111.03	4.03	27.56		
Mode	Hypothesis	21.10	1.00	21.10	68.46	0.0
	Error	2.54	8.24	0.31		
User	Hypothesis	126.25	4.00	31.56	130.05	0.0
	Error	0.97	4.00	0.24		
Mode * User	Hypothesis	0.97	4.00	0.24	0.32	0.86
	Error	19.50	26.00	0.75		

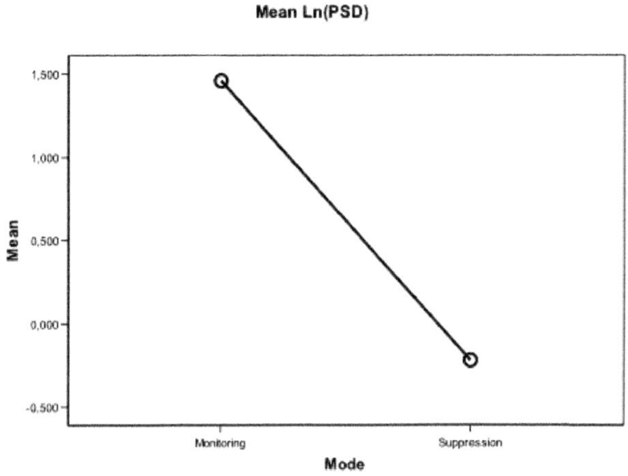

Fig. 5.5 Mode effect on the Ln(PSD)

The results also indicated that the range of reduction in tremor energy for signals above this orthosis operational limit ranges from 3.4 % (percentile 5) to 95.2 % (percentile 95) in relation to energy in monitoring mode.

These reductions can be appreciated in figure 5.7 and figure 5.8. These figures illustrate the effects of WOTAS on tremorous movement using both strategies. Figure 5.7 illustrates the time series corresponding to the tremorous movement of the elbow joint of user 2 while the arm is outstretched. The top part of the figure shows the time signal with WOTAS in the *monitoring* mode. Notice that for both *passive* and *active modes* the amplitude of tremor is clearly smaller than in the *monitoring mode*.

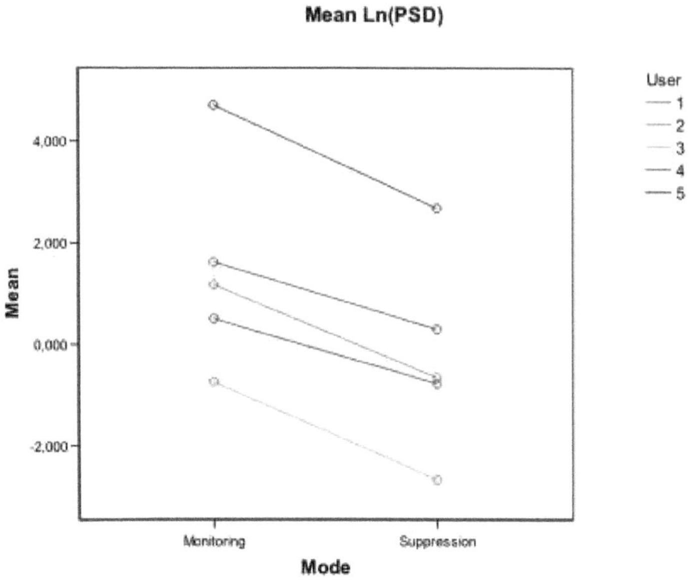

Fig. 5.6 Effect of the user in the reduction of tremor with WOTAS.

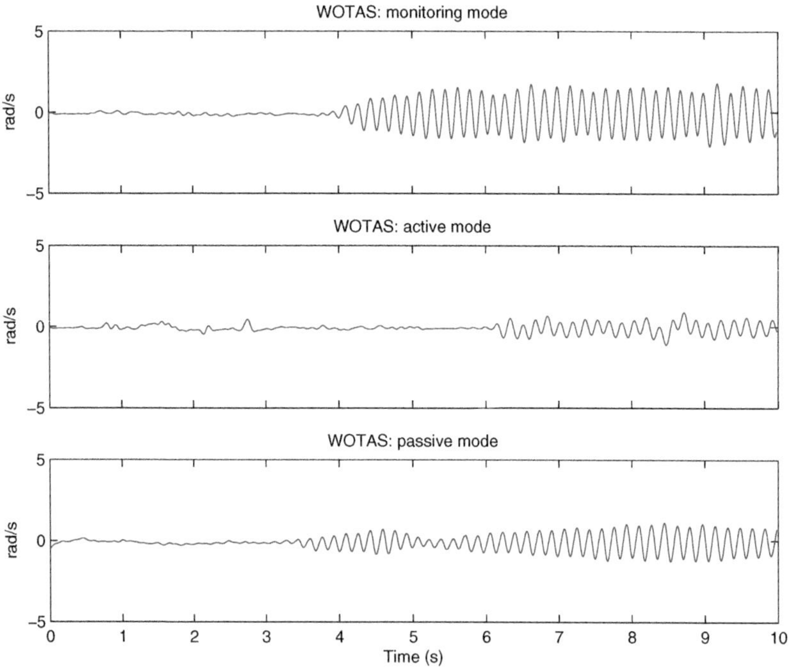

Fig. 5.7 This figure illustrates the oscillations of the elbow of tremor with WOTAS in a monitoring mode and suppressing modes in user 2. Note the strong reduction in amplitude of tremor when suppressing actions are applied. Oscillations are expressed in rad/sec.

Figure 5.8 illustrates the same reduction in the frequency domain. The Power Spectrum Density (PSD) have been obtained from the part of the signal with tremor. The top part of the figure illustrates the PSD of the tremorous movement with WOTAS operating in *monitoring* mode. It is possible to see a clear peak of tremor activity close to 4 Hz. In the middle, figure shows the PSD while WOTAS was operating in active mode. Notice that the energy associated to tremor activity has been substantially reduced. In the low part of the figure the peak of energy corresponding to the tremorous activity when WOTAS is in passive mode also presents a clear reduction. These results indicate that WOTAS is able to suppress tremor in addition to validate both control strategies proposed, active and passive, for control of orthotic suppression of tremor. Notice that the frequency of tremor does not change when the exoskeleton is working in suppression modes.

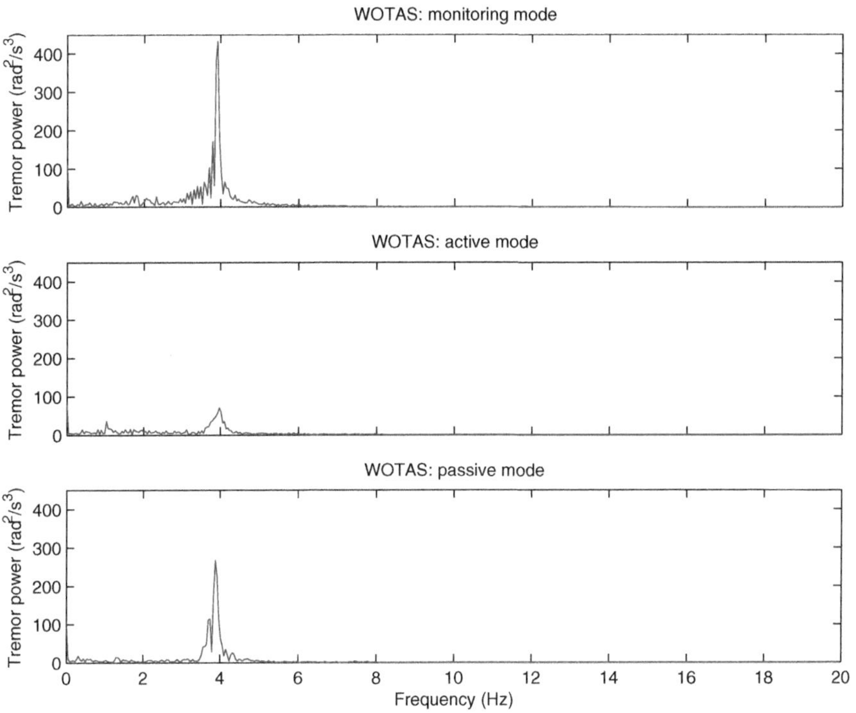

Fig. 5.8 This figure illustrates the associated power spectral density (PSD) of tremor WOTAS in a monitoring mode (upper part) and suppressing modes in user 2. Notice the strong reduction in the PSD of tremor when suppressing actions are applied. PSD is expressed in $\frac{rad^2}{s^3}$.

A detailed analysis of the data showed that the active suppression strategy (81.2 % mean power reduction) presents higher levels of tremor suppression compared to passive suppression strategy (70 % mean power reduction), see figure 5.9 . This suggests a better performance of the active mode in tremor suppression.

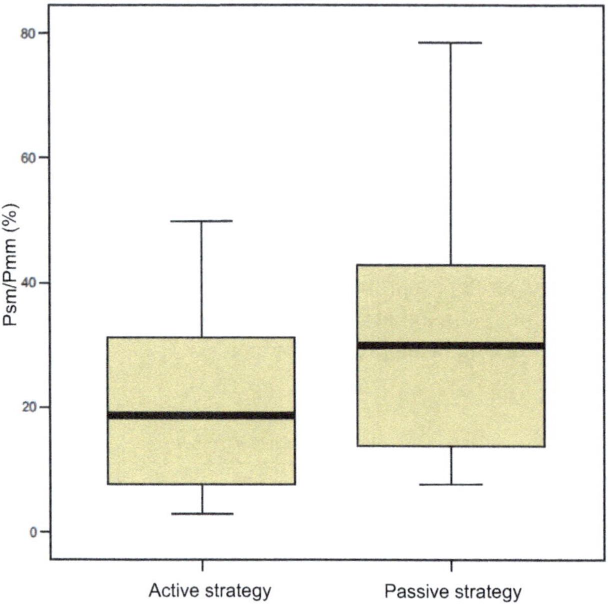

Fig. 5.9 Comparison of the tremor suppression results obtained with both control strategies. *Left:* active control strategy and *Right:* passive control strategy.

Nevertheless, we consider that this difference is not statistics meaningful. We believe that experiments with more patients should be performed in order to clearly evaluate the performance of both strategies. This is due to the fact that during these experiments the viscosity added to the different joint movements (elbow and wirst flexion-extension and forearm pronation-supination) was the same. Further experiments should be performed with customized biomechanical parameters according to the particular biomechanical properties of each user, [92]. This solution was considered during the validation phase; nevertheless it could not be implemented in order to maintain the experimental duration smaller than 1 hour, [13].

As to the subjective evaluation, patients reported that they prefer the passive strategy instead of the active one. We believe that this is because when operating in the active mode, the exoskeleton is constantly moving out-of-phase to tremor, which could be more unpleasant to the user. Moreover, this generates more acoustic noise, which could be more disagreeable to the user.

5.3 Discussion

The previous section presents results of the clinical trials related to the evaluation of the exoskeleton for tremor suppression presented in the paper. The exoskeleton performance was assessed in 10 users suffering from different kinds of tremors at the upper-limb. Two strategies for tremor reduction have been tested: viscous friction and notch filtering.

The analysis of the videos from the experiments demonstrated that in the majority of users there was no tremor displacement to proximal joints of the upper limb. Nevertheless, one user in ten presented an increment in tremor activity at shoulder level. The authors believe that future work should be performed in order to investigate and define the profile of the users affected by this phenomenon.

The results of the experiments indicated that the device could achieve a consistent 40% of tremor power reduction for all users, being able to attain a reduction ratio in the order of 80% tremor power in specific joints of users with severe tremor. In addition, the users reported that the exoskeleton did not affect their voluntary motion. These results indicate the feasibility of tremor suppression through biomechanical loading. Nevertheless, the users reported that the exoskeleton could not be considered as a solution to their problem since it is bulky and heavy. The users considered that the use of such device should cause social exclusion. This was expected since the exoskeleton was developed as a platform to evaluate the concept of mechanical tremor suppression and not as a final orthotic solution. The main wish expressed by the potential users was the possibility of hiding the exoskeleton under clothing, [114].

The results also indicated a superior performance of active tremor suppression over passive tremor suppression. However, the authors believe that this could be due to the fact that the value of viscosity added to the movement was the same for all users. The customization of viscosity or inertia added to the upper limb according to the biomechanical characteristics of each user should improve the efficiency of passive tremor suppression strategy, [92, 114].

It was noticed that the degree of tremor reduction was dependent upon the power associated with tremor. There are lower limits for robotic tremor suppression that should be determined for the mechanical impedance of the contact exoskeleton-skin, and the particular morphology of tremor.

Another important aspect of this validation is that the physical interaction affects the cognitive interaction between the robot and the human. In general, physical HR interaction will trigger cognitive processes on either side of the HR interface. These cognitive processes will in turn affect motor control both in the human and in the robot, all in a context of mutual adaptation during interaction. This adaptation mechanism has not been clearly formalized in the literature, most probably due to the complexity of the CNS and related motor control mechanisms, [95].

During the trials two users spontaneously reported that they felt a decrease in the amplitude of their tremorous movement and consequently they felt more confident about the execution of the task. This indicates that the visual feedback of a smooth movement has a positive impact in the user. This fact is very important and future research will be performed in order to evaluate this phenomenon with more users of different pathologies.

When tremor is counteracted by the interaction between human and robot, the following phenomena are observed:

1. The visual feedback of a limb with a reduced tremor amplitude has a positive impact on the human control system. The human motor control is reinforced (a sort of positive gain feedback), and residual tremor is further reduced as a result.

2. The reduction of tremor in one joint following interaction with the robot results in perturbed human motor control, possibly leading to increased tremor intensity at the adjacent proximal joints. This phenomenon is called Distal to Proximal Tremor Shift (DPTS).

Two adaptive control strategies, impedance control (see section 4.4.1) and model-based repetitive control (see section 4.4.2), were proposed. As described in chapter 4, the following approach was adopted to manage both of the physically triggered human motor control phenomena.

1. The control strategies exhibit an adaptive behaviour. In the case of impedance control, the combined impedance of each articulation of the HR system is calculated on the basis of a real-time estimation of the tremor amplitude. In the case of repetitive control, the amplitude of the force applied to counteract tremor is also based on the continuous estimation and tracking of tremor frequency and amplitude. Thus the system can respond to the changes that take place in the human motor system. The outcome of the adaptive approach to both control strategies is mutual adaptation, both physical and cognitive.
2. The implementation of the control strategies is based on individual independent control loops in each joint of the exoskeleton. This minimizes the DPTS problem: if cancellation of the tremor in one joint increases the tremor in the other joint, the algorithm responsible for controlling the adjacent joint will automatically identify the increased tremor and try to reduce the tremor migration. The aim is to achieve equilibrium between the active behaviour of tremor reduction in either joint, thereby reducing the coupling effects of the upper-limb joints.

Based on the result, authors could claim that their approach in the development of the control strategies was succesful.

5.4 Conclusions

This chapter presented the validation of a robotic exoskeleton able to monitor, diagnose and control tremor in subjects. The exoskeleton was evaluated with 10 users and validated the concept of tremor suppression through wearable robotics. Both proposed strategies for tremor suppression (viscous friction and notch-filtering) have produced significant reduction of tremor amplitude. The results indicated that notch-filtering of tremor is more efficient than viscous friction, however further research should be performed in order to validate this statement.

Some aspects of mechanical tremor suppression were not evaluated in this study, further trials with a larger number of users should be held in order to evaluate other different aspects of WOTAS operation. The exoskeleton will help to analyze the effect of biomechanical loading on the upper limb motion and quantify its effects on fatigue. In addition, the carryover of attenuation effects after the impedance is removed must be subject to study. This is in line with the study of the effects of long term strengthening of muscles when subject to the training effect the exoskeleton is imposing to the user.

Another very important issue is the interface of the exoskeleton with the upper limb. It was detected that there are lower limits for robotic tremor suppression determined by the mechanical impedance of the contact exoskeleton-upper limb. These limitations make the device useless for users with moderate to low tremor. There are several biomechanical aspects regarding the transmission of forces from the actuators to the limb that should be solved in order to improve the exoskeleton performance. Another aspect that requires further research is the effect of visual feedback on the capacity of the user to perform a task.

In this work, the use of biomechanical loading (by means of orthotic exoskeletons), both technically and clinically, as a new method for tremor suppression with successful results. The device was clinically validated with tremor patients (from different pathologies: essential tremor, Parkinson, Multiple sclerosis, Post-traumatic tremor and mixed tremor) with successful results: it was able to achieve a consistent 40 % of tremor power reduction for all patients, and to attain a reduction ratio in the order of 80 % tremor power in specific joints of patients with severe tremor. Moreover, patients related that the exoskeleton did not affect their concomitant voluntary motion, which is a common drawback of tremor and very important for users acceptance.

Results indicated that the approach to mechanical suppression of tremor by means of orthotic devices presents limitations mainly due to the physical interaction between the exoskeleton and the human limb:

- The transmission of forces through soft tissues plays an important role in the efficiency of tremor suppression. There is a physical limitation for tremor suppression through wearable devices due to force generation (size and power consumption of the actuators) and transmission through soft tissues.
- Emerging actuators technologies, i.e. Magneto-Rheological Fluid actuators (MRFs), Electro-Active Polymer actuators (EAP) and Ultrasonic motors, were evaluated for an orthotic implementation [14]. It was concluded that, despite the success of the approach, there is no suitable actuator technology in terms of cosmetic and aesthetic (low weight, compact to be worn beneath the clothes) as well as functional requirements (torque, bandwidth), [94].
- Patients related that these bulky exoskeletons could not be considered as a solution to their problem since it is considered that the use of such device should cause social exclusion.

In summary, robotics based solutions have shown clinical evidence of the approach based on human limb impedance control. However it results in bulky and non cosmetic solutions for which patients are especially reluctant.

Chapter 6
Summary, Conclusions and Upcoming Research

6.1 Summary

This book started with an introduction to Rehabilitation Robotics and, in particular, of Rehabilitation Wearable Robots of which Exoskeletons are very interesting examples. A historical note that dated back to the late 1960's the first work on Rehabilitation Robotics was given in Chapter 1. Even though this represents already more than 40 years of work in the area, when looking to publications and scientific contributions in the field, one might say that it is still in its infancy.

The first chapter highlighted the salient aspects of Exoskeletons and Rehabilitation Robotics. These devices can only be fully understood when considered biomechatronic devices. This is mainly due to the close interaction of these devices with the human user and to the use of nature and human biology as a source of inspiration when designing Exoskeletons.

The close human–robot interaction was split in chapter 1 into cognitive and physical interaction. Both are equally important in exoskeletons but the physical interaction leads to strict demands on safety and dependability. On the other hand, as physical interaction is in most instances triggered by a cognitive interaction, also strict demands on reliability, accuracy and robustness are derived to the cognitive interface.

This book addressed the design and evaluation of a wearable exoskeleton to suppress pathological tremor. Tremor is a rhythmic involuntary movement of human limbs that can lead to disability. Being tremor the focus of this book, chapter 2 was devoted to thoroughly studying how tremor affect limbs at joint level. This has been considered crucial as the approach adopted in the framework of this research was to use an exoskeleton working on the internal force concept. This implies that forces are applied to the human skeletal structure through soft tissues between members in a limb, e.g. between forearm and arm to suppress tremor in the elbow.

By adopting the internal force concept, tremors appearing in joints not spanned by the exoskeleton cannot be suppressed. This might be considered a drawback but has the advantage of allowing lighter and more compact robotic exoskeletal structures, and therefore wearability can be a realistic target. Having tis in mind,

E. Rocon and J.L. Pons: Exoskeletons in Rehabilitation Robotics, STAR 69, pp. 113–130.
springerlink.com

chapter 2 analyzed tremor characteristics in the most relevant tremor groups, i.e. rest tremors (Parkinson's disease), postural tremors (essential tremor) and intention tremor. These characteristics included tremor patterns, tremor torque and power for the most relevant joints contributing to disabling hand tremors. It was concluded that elbow flexion–extension, forearm abduction–adduction and wrist flexion–extension need to be considered for an efficient tremor suppression exoskeletal approach.

Tremor characterization at joint level was the starting point for the design and selection of technologies. Tremor characterization was based on a biomechanical model of the human upper limb and on especially designed signal processing tools for an efficient capture of the non-stationary characteristics of tremor. Kinematic and dynamic analysis tools as typically used in the context of studying artificial kinematic chains, e.g. robotic manipulators, were used to model upper limb kinematics and dynamics. Empirical mode decomposition (EMD) and the Hilbert spectrum were adopted and adapted to analyze tremor.

Once tremor is understood and the effects of tremor on joints and limbs quantified, the rest of the book adopted a structure in which the importance of both the cognitive HR interaction (cHRI) and the physical HR interaction (pHRI) was highlighted. Chapter 3 was devoted to explain the approach to develop the cognitive interaction between the robotic exoskeletal structure and the human.

Typically, a cognitive human–robot interface has the goal of decoding and transmitting volitional commands from the user to the robot and grasping relevant parameters of the robot-environment interaction to be fed back to the user. In our case, the cognitive human robot interaction scheme is rather unusual. The main goal of the cognitive interface is not deciphering volitional command but identifying tremor onset and tremor characteristics over time as it is only when tremor is present when the robotics exoskeletal structure has to apply tremor suppression mechanisms. In this context, the goal is detecting whether the user is trembling or not and, in case its is being affected by tremor, to track tremor characteristics, e.g. joints affected, tremor amplitude, tremor frequency.

Once the cognitive HRI was introduced and discussed in chapter 3, the exoskeletal WOTAS system together with the tremor suppression control strategies were introduced in Chapter 4. As already above mentioned, dependability and safety in exskeletons depends to a great extent on the quality of the physical HRI. In this chapter all aspects in relation to this physical interaction were addressed. We started by biomechanically modelling the upper limb as a previous step to ensure safe application of load through soft tissues. Since we adopted the internal force concept in the design of WOTAS, carefull consideration of force transmission through soft tissues is a must. This modelling approach was also complemented by an in-depth analysis of user's tolerance to pressure. In this regard, maps showing users' tolerance to pressure and shear forces were derived and then used to design supports.

All mechatronics foundations for the design of WOTAS were also addressed in chapter 4. In particular, a full section was devoted to introduce the mechacical design of the system, the selection of sensing technologies and, more importantly, the choice of actuator technologies. The analysis of the mechanical design of WOTAS highlighted the need of developing full kinematic compatibility between the exoskeletal structure and the anatomical joints being spanned by the robot. This was easily achievable in the case of both elbow and wrist flexion-extension DoFs, but it was much more complex in the case of forearm pronation and supination. In this particular case, a redundant kinematic chain comprising revolute, universal and linear joints was used to ensure kinematic compatibility.

Actuators (and the accompanying power technologies) have always been a bottleneck when fully wearable robotics technologies have been considered. In this book different novel alternatives have been addressed but it was already in 1982, in the framework of a workshop held at MIT, [58], where it was pointed out the current actuator technologies are the most serious, long term impediment to the development of artificial hands. Artificial hands are only an example application of wearable robots, therefore the same limitations apply to other robots and, in particular, to WOTAS.

During these two decades Shape Memory Alloys have been studied as a possible actuator technology, but efficiency, reliability and response time are claimed as the most limiting factors. On the other hand, high torque ultrasonic motors were also proposed as alternative technologies. Again, efficiency and high voltages required for operation are the main drawbacks even when the choice is more balanced as compared to traditional EM motors, [94]. Here, both Ultrasonic motors and traditional DC EM motors have been considered. Last generation Ultrasonic motors looked promising but control problems, especially when being driven at low velocities, favoured the selection of traditional, reliable EM motors. This of course resulted in bulky solutions but gave us the flexibility to implement several control strategies to suppress tremor and eventually, allowed the validation of the concept.

Two tremor suppression control strategies were introduced in Chapter 4. Both tremor suppression strategies are based on the peculiar rhythmic characteristics of tremor and on the mechanical behaviour of human limbs and joints. The first tremor suppression control approach, the so-called active strategy, is a repetitive, model based control approach. It is imported from noise cancellation applications where out-of-phase noise is additively applied so that overall noise is cancelled. In our case, tremor is detected and identified at each joint level and then the limb is driven with an out-of-phase tremor at the same frequency and amplitude that pathological tremor. It was estimated that a small phase lag, i.e. around 20-30 ms, would result in uncomfortable sensations and even amplified tremor. As a consequence, strict requirements in terms of real time implementation of the cognitive interface algorithms (to detect and track tremor characteristics) and control strategies were derived.

The second tremor suppression strategy is based on the second order characteristics of the human upper limb joints. It was shown that human limbs can be modelled as second order linear systems. Mechanically, human joints behave as low pass filters. Here we identified that most volitional movements occur below 2 Hz while for most tremors, typical frequencies are in the order of 3–12 Hz. Therefore, if the stiffness, damping and inertia of a human limb' s joint are tuned so that the cut-off frequency of the equivalent mechanical system lay below the tremor frequency and above the volitional movement range, the human limb should naturally filter out tremor while preserving voluntary movements. This is exactly the approach we implemented as our second tremor suppression strategy.

Finally, Chapter 5 was devoted to the validation and proof of concept of the hypothesis: tremor can be effectively managed by means of exoskeletal loading the upper limb. In this regard, this chapter introduced the experimental protocol specifically designed to this end. In short, a double-blind protocol was designed with provisions to consider possible *placebo effect* when using the tremor suppression exoskeleton. Potential users representing all main tremor groups were included in the pre-clinical trials but, in the sample, patients exhibiting postural tremor were over represented. This was expressely done in view of the fact that this tremor group is the one that will most benefit of a mechanical tremor suppression management.

6.2 Conclusions

A detailed presentation of results and the subsequent discussion was already given in chapter 5, only a few considerations will be given here. It is worth stressing that, upon application of tremor reduction strategies by means of WOTAS, the best results were observed in patients exhibiting severe tremors whilst those being affected by mild or light tremors only underwent slight tremor reductions or, in the worst cases, even tremor amplification. This was explained in terms of *bad transmission of (low) cancelling forces through forearm and arm soft tissues.*

It is also important to note that the cognitive HRI interaction in this particular application is only based on the analysis of limb movement. This has implications that need to be clarified. On the one hand, this means that *tremor can only be detected and tracked when upper limbs are already trembling*. Therefore, tremor cancellation strategies can only act after allowing a first period of tremor which, in some instances, is undesirable. On the other hand, other sources of information on tremor are not considered. Limb movement in humans is a mechanism that involve central and peripheral structures. Voluntary movement is planned at brain level, this motor planning is then coordinated by means of brain, spinal and peripheral mechanisms. All this process results in electrical activity (EMG) stimulating muscles. When tremor is present, this is a result of involuntary oscillators at brain level which lead to undesired rhythmic EMG activity. If all these steps in motor planning and execution are considered in a cognitive HRI a priori (before it actually happens) knowledge of trembling movement can be derived. *This leads to the need of proposing multimodal cognitive HRI schemes where all stages in motor mechanisms are considered.*

WOTAS has been subjectively evaluated by all patients participating in preclinical trials. The overall degree of satisfaction with tremor reduction results was high. However *all patients reported issues related to the usability* of a solution like WOTAS. Functionally the system is very well perceived but it is bulky, noisy and energy consumption is a concern for a truly wearable solution. Therefore, from a usability standpoint, we are still far from an ideal solution.

6.3 Upcoming Research

Tremor cancellation, as proposed in this book, can only be understood in the general context of restoring human motor function in the widest scope. Restoring human motor functions has been a fascinating yet frustrating research area during the last century. The possibility of interfacing the human nervous system with mechatronic devices, and then employ these devices to restore neurological function, has long fascinated scientists, [23]. The paradigmatic scenario for technological restoration of sensory and motor function is Spinal Cord Injury (SCI), where flow of sensory and motor neural information is interrupted following a partial or total medullar lesion. However, other frequent neural disorders, e.g. tremor as in this book or Cerebrovascular Accidents (CVA) and Cerebral Palsy (CP), would benefit from these rehabilitation or functional compensation systems.

First instances of Rehabilitation Robots (RRs) were industrial robots adapted and brought to the rehabilitation environment, [26]-[22]. The adoption of industrial robots in rehabilitation settings immediately led to issues in terms of acceptability, usability, safety and dependability. In this context, the concept of Wearable Robots (WRs) was proposed by Pons, [95]. Wearable robots are person-oriented robots and therefore more adapted to the interaction with users. They are worn by human operators to supplement the function of a limb, e.g. exoskeletons. WRs exhibit a close interaction with the human user but structurally are similar to robots, i.e. rigid links, actuators, sensors and control electronics.

The next step in robot-assisted rehabilitation leads to the concept of Soft Robots (SRs). They are also wearable, but SRs use functional human structures instead of artificial counterparts, e.g. artificial actuators are substituted by Functional Electrical Stimulation (FES) of human muscles. The borderline between human and robot becomes fuzzy and this immediately leads to hybrid Human-Robot systems.

It is in this context that Neurorobots (NRs) and Motor Neuroprostheses (MNPs) emerge. Both seek to obtain motor command signals from motor control regions of the nervous system via Brain-Machine interfaces (BMIs).

MNPs constitute an approach to restoring function by means of artificially controlling human muscles or muscle nerves with Functional Electrical Stimulation (FES). MNPs are shown in figure 6.1 as a bypass of damaged sensory-motor systems: users volitionally (via a BMI) trigger delivery of electrical stimulation by using the functional part of the body (above lesion); Electrical pulses stimulate motor and/or sensory nerves, thereby generating movement by activating paralyzed muscles.

Pioneering work in multichannel FES with surface electrodes was done by a research group from Ljubljana, Slovenia, [134]. They developed a three-channel system for assisting the swing phase in individuals with hemiplegia. Vienna FES system, [16], Compex Motion, [97], and UNA FET, [98], are examples of state-of-the-art multichannel transcutaneous systems that can be used for gait restoration in individuals with hemiplegia or paraplegia.

In order to overcome deficiencies of the surface systems (e.g., donning and doffing, proper electrode placement, poor stimulation selectivity), a number of

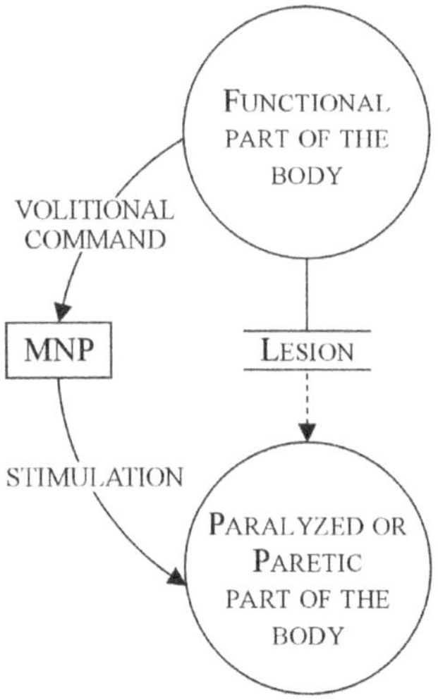

Fig. 6.1 Scheme of a MNPs.

percutaneous and implanted systems were suggested. However, implantable FES systems suffer from adverse reactions of the human immune system that prevent long term and permanent solutions, energy supply to implanted systems is not properly solved (even though wireless inductive systems seem promising), difficult heat dissipation and wiring issues.

Human body is a highly complex musculoskeletal system. However, FES control patterns to drive, for instance, human lower limbs during MNP walking, are very simple and use control signals that are rather coarse. Therefore, it is not surprising that gait patterns generated by using contemporary MNPs are still far from the performances typical for normal gait of able-bodied individuals. The movements are rather jerky. Walking is frequently accompanied with significant energy expenditure and high heart rates and, in addition, FES typically results in pain and muscle fatigue.

NRs use volitional commands for controlling a (mechatronic) WR (typically an exoskeleton, as in the case of WOTAS in this book) which, in turn, applies controlled forces to drive paralyzed limbs. This approach is schematically depicted in figure 6.2. Wearable Neurorobotics is more versatile as to the implementation of motor actions: (1) precise kinematics and impedance control is readily available, (2) biomimetic control architectures, e.g. Central Pattern Generators (CPGs), internal models (model-based feed-forward control) and reflexes, can be readily applied, and (3) built-in artificial proprioception (limb awareness) and vestibular sensors can be used to drive non-volitional motor actions, e.g. control of balance. As a serious drawback, the transmission of motor actions (forces) to the human musculoskeletal system takes place through soft tissues.

In NRs, the interaction is to be carefully thought in terms of compatible kinematics and application of controlled forces. Moreover, current limitations in efficient

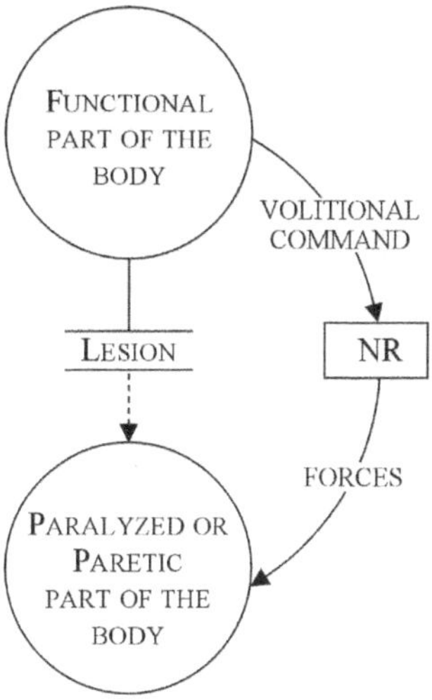

Fig. 6.2 Scheme of NRs: functional compensation is attained by application of restoring forces by an exoskeleton.

and compact artificial actuator technologies, as pointed out by Pons, [94], suggest NP alternatives, e.g. FES.

The common component in MNPs and NRs is a BMI to decipher volitional commands from the user as input for the MNP and NR controllers. As to BMIs, current trends lead to integrating brain activity (electroencephalography, EEG and other invasive and non-invasive sources), neural activity (ENG), neuromuscular activity (EMG) and limb motion for robusts interfaces [95]. It is accepted that, for Real-Time (RT) control of NRs or MNPs, current non-invasive brain-machine interface (BMI) technology is a limiting factor. However, as in implantable FES electrodes, invasive and implantable cortical or peripheral electrodes elicit glial reactions, thus become non-functional in the medium to long term.

It is accepted that, if invasive techniques are set aside, control of NPs and NRs requires mimicking human neuromotor system in which decentralised mechanisms (CPGs, reflexes, control of balance) are implemented to alleviate RT control requirements on the non-invasive BMI. As an example, a model for gait should contain the mechanisms located in the spinal cord: (1) the reflexes mediated by the muscle spindles, the Golgi Tendon Organs and the skin receptors, and (2) the CPGs modelled by means of half-centre non-linear oscillators. All of these circuits act as decentralised mechanisms but have inhibiting or facilitating inputs from higher centres. If a model of how these and other mechanisms are orchestrated by the human neuromotor system is obtained, it would be possible to: (1) integrate them in the control architecture of a MNP or NR system thus alleviating the requirements on volitional control; and (2) analyse the sensitivity of the movement patterns fed to the musculoskeletal system to each one of these control mechanisms and derive clinical value of these models.

In a recent 3-day scientific meeting on advances in neural rehabilitation engineering[1] (in which the authors of this book actively participated) the international context in the research field of neural rehabilitation was thoroughly analysed. The consensus indicated that the above stated limitations and shortcomings of MNPs and NRs for neural rehabilitation are still actual.

Motor Neuroprosthetics and Neurorobotics is a very active scientific area involving numerous disciplines. The field is actively supported by US, Japan and EU administrations. Just to mention our closest research environment, MNP and NR are supported by EU FP7 in a number of programmes, e.g. the Virtual Physiological Human programme of eHealth, ICT (Cognitive Systems and Robotics as well as eInclusion), and FET Proactive (Brain-Inspired ICT and Human-Computer Confluence):

- The European Future and Emerging Technologies (FET) research scheme launched the first European research projects on information systems inspired by biology and neuroscience. Expected impacts of MNP-NR research, extending well beyond ICT, include novel technology based on non-invasive BMIs that empower/assist handicapped persons[2] .
- Coordinated research on MNP-NR restoration of human motor function will aim at building up critical mass and integrating (until now) fragmented research efforts. The recently launched Virtual Physiological Human (VPH) project and the Blue Brain project[3] illustrate the relevance of such endeavours, at international level[4].
- In the framework of restoring human function by means of MNPs and NRs, research on novel ideas that overcome current limitations in neural rehabilitation will show up. In order to do this, the understanding of information processing in biological systems leading to artificial systems that can be naturally combined with biological systems (such as bidirectional brain/machine interfacing), in accordance to the European ICT research agenda, e.g. Bio-ICT convergence[5], need to be addressed.

---

[1] Symposium on Advances in Neural Rehabilitation Engineering, August 23-25, 2010. Center for Sensory-Motor Interaction (SMI), Aalborg University.

[2] FET is characterized by high-risk builds on synergies and cross-fertilisation between different disciplines such as biology, nano-, neuro- and cognitive science, ethology or social science or economics.

[3] Blue Brain is the first comprehensive attempt to reverse-engineer the mammalian brain, in order to understand brain function and dysfunction with the aid of detailed simulations. http://bluebrain.epfl.ch/

[4] VPH aims at personalised simulation of the human body, promising unprecedented progress in disease prevention and healthcare. It combines efforts across the Framework Programme with global cooperation, in particular with the USA. http://www.vph-noe.eu/

[5] FP7 FET Proactive Initiative.

In this context future research activities will aim at:

1. restoring motor function in patients with neurological conditions (tremor, SCI, CVA, CP and other) through an integrated application of NRs and MNPs in a functional compensation approach; and
2. promoting motor control re-learning in patients suffering all these conditions by means of an integrated use of NRs and MNPs.

A new and unconventional approach is required. Motor control of human limbs during manipulation and locomotion will be the result of three systems acting mechanically in parallel, see figure 6.3:

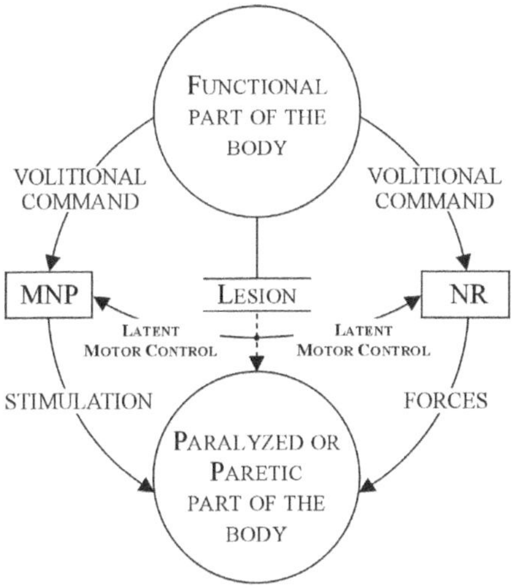

Fig. 6.3 The latent human capabilities are prioritised, only when weakness in human motor control is perceived the actions of a MNP and a NR are orchestrated.

1. the biological system through the latent motor capabilities of the patients,
2. the motor control of human limbs by means of the MNP, and
3. the motor control of human limbs by means of a light and wearable NR.

The *Assist-as-Needed paradigm* is assumed, which accounts for the variability in the human neuromuscular structures, an intrinsic property of neuromuscular control. Thus, the parallel actuation (NR-MNP) is not fixed but dynamically adapted and subject to the changes due to neural organizations and muscular adaptations.

This approach will promote both sensory and motor control re-training and brain plasticity thus leading to rehabilitation and functional compensation solutions for Tremor, SCI, CVA and CP patients amongst others.

In order to meet this ambitious aim, the following partial objectives need to be addressed:

- To develop: (1) an accurate engineering model of the human musculoskeletal system (both upper and lower limbs) for a safe and efficient application of FES by the MNP and (2) an accurate engineering model of human anatomy (joints both of upper and lower limbs) and soft tissues for a safe and efficient transmission of forces from the NR to the user.
- To develop engineering models of the human neuromotor mechanisms being implemented in control of walking, standing, reaching and grasping in healthy humans.
- To develop a control structure and algorithms mimicking the biological model for an efficient and safe orchestration of the three actors: (1) human latent characteristics, (2) MNP and (3) NR. This need to be particularised for each application scenario.
- To develop actuator, sensor and energy management technologies so that the NR-MNP can be embodied in a portable, ambulatory, usable and acceptable solution for the patient and the therapist.
- To develop a multimodal Brain and Neural to Machine interface (BNMI) capable of deciphering volitional commands in a robust manner. This also involves handling undesired motion, e.g. spasm or tremors, and assessing human latent capability.
- To elicit patients and therapists requirements for an acceptable solution and to provide means for patient engagement and validation of the systems.

All these research activities are ongoing at the Bioengineering Group, CSIC. They are part of a large-scale project called HYPER[6] which is funded by CONSOLIDER-INGENIO programme of the Spanish Ministry of Science and Innovation. The HYPER project intends to represent a breakthrough in the research of neurorobotic (NR) and motor neuroprosthetic (MNP) devices in close cooperation with the human body, both for rehabilitation and functional compensation of motor disorders in activities of daily living.

However in the particular scenario of tremor suppression ongoing research activities are being carried out in the framework of the European project TREMOR[7]. The main objective of the project is to validate, technically, functionally and clinically, the concept of mechanically suppressing tremor through selective Functional Electrical Stimulation (FES) based on a (Brain-to-Computer Interaction) BCI-driven detection of involuntary (tremor) motor activity:

- The system will detect and monitor involuntary motor activity (tremor) through a multimodal BCI. The proposed BCI will combine CNS (Electroencephalography, EEG) and PNS (Electromyography, EMG) data with biomechanical data

[6] Research supported by CONSOLIDER-INGENIO 2010 Programme of the Spanish Ministry of Science and Innovation, (grant CSD2009-00067).
[7] Research supported by FP7 project TREMOR (ICT2007-224051).

(Inertial Measurement Units, IMUs) in a sensor fusion approach. It will model and track tremor and voluntary motion.

- It will also include a multi-channel array FES system for selective stimulation of muscles for tremor suppression while reducing the influence on voluntary motion.
- For a satisfactory usability the embodiment must fit potential user expectations in terms of cosmetics, functionality and aesthetics.

TREMOR proposes a multimodal BCI in which the main goal is identifying, characterizing and tracking involuntary motor bioelectrical activity as a command to trigger a biomechanical suppression of tremor. Therefore it follows the general scheme of MNP-NR management of motor disorder as set forth in the objectives of HYPER.

The TREMOR robot takes the form of an active garment (sleeve) that incoporates sewed electrodes on both electrical stimulation and recording, beign a garment-based embodiment totally wearable and compatible with normal human clothes. As all wearable robots, the major characteristic of the TREMOR neurorobot is its strong interaction with the user, [95]. This interaction is both physical and cognitive, and happens in a bidirectional manner. In our case, the cognitive Human–Robot Interface (cHRI) is built upon a BNCI that assesses the generation, transmission, and execution of both voluntary and tremorous movements. On the other hand, the physical Human–Robot Interface (pHRI) comprises a multichannel FES system that selectively drives the muscles based on the output of the control algorithm. The TREMOR neurorobot takes the shape of an active garment (a sleeve) that incorporates arrays of sewn electrodes for both electrical stimulation and recording, aiming at satisfying users aesthetical' preferences and usuability requirements. Moreover, stimulation through electrode matrices allows us to implement techniques to minimize fatigue, discomfort and painful sensations, [96], at the same time that we enhance the selectivity of the simulation.

The BNCI comprises recording of electroencephalographic (EEG) and electromyographic (EMG) activity, together with motion capture with inertial measurement units (IMUs). Each sensor modality aims at extracting certain information, following a hierarchical integration scheme, i.e. one modality activates the other, Figure 6.4. First, a real–time EEG classifier is in charge of detecting user's intention to perform a voluntary movement, waking up the system. Next, processing of sEMG information yields tremor onset and an estimation of its frequency. Finally, IMUs track instantaneous tremor amplitude and frequency at each joint. FES based tremor suppression will be driven by instantaneous tremor parameters provided by IMUs. The use of multiple sensor modalities also permits us implementing fusion and redundancy techniques to enhance the dependability of the system. One example of redundancy is the use of EMG activity to detect the occurence of a motor command, compensating for eventual EEG classification errors. An example of sensor fusion is the use of machine learning techniques to adjust the parameters of the EEG clasisifier after the execution of a movement, as detected with IMUs.

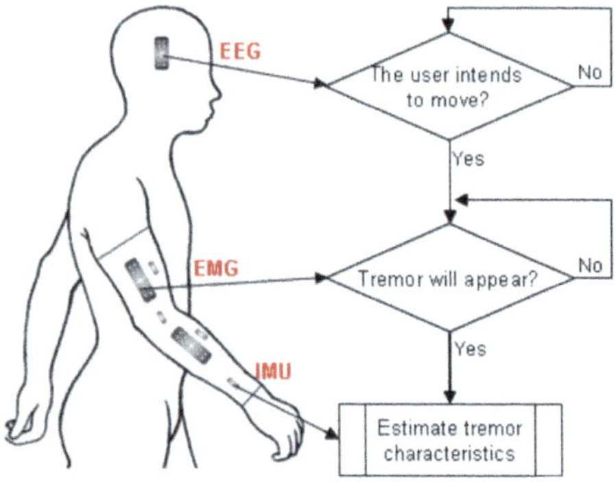

Fig. 6.4 Integration of sensor modalities to drive FES based tremor suppression. First, EEG monitors if the user intends to perform a voluntary motion. Once this has been detected, tremor onset is derived from EMG information . Finally, after the system detects tremor will appear, tremor parameters are tracked based on IMUs.

The physical interface of this soft wearable robot aims at taking advantage of biomechanical loading as a selective means for compensating for tremor. Hence, the system will filter out the tremor, leaving concomitant voluntary motion unaltered, based on the application of FES through an array of textile electrodes. Command signals to drive the stimulators are provided by a control strategy that relies on the information of the BNCI described above, and on an inverse dynamic model of the musculoskeletal system.

The soft wearable robot described above has been implemented as an experimental platform that comprises both the BNCI and the multichannel FES system, interfacing with the user through the soft robot. A master computer running Neutrino RealTime Operating System (QNX Software Systems, Ontario, Canada) is in charge of synchronizing and integrating the information from the different sensor modalities, and driving the FES units. This platform has been built and validated with patients in an iterative fashion, and in its current form comprises the following systems: 1) a 16 channel EEG amplifier (gUSBamp, Guger Technologies OG), 2) a 128 channel surface EMG amplifier (EMG-USB, OT Bioelettronica), 3) a motion capture system based on IMUs (TechMCS, Technaid SL), 4) multichannel, individually controllable, electrical stimulators (Tremuna, UNA Systems), and 5) an smart textile (SMARTEX). Figure 6.5 shows a control subject wearing the conceptual TREMOR robot.

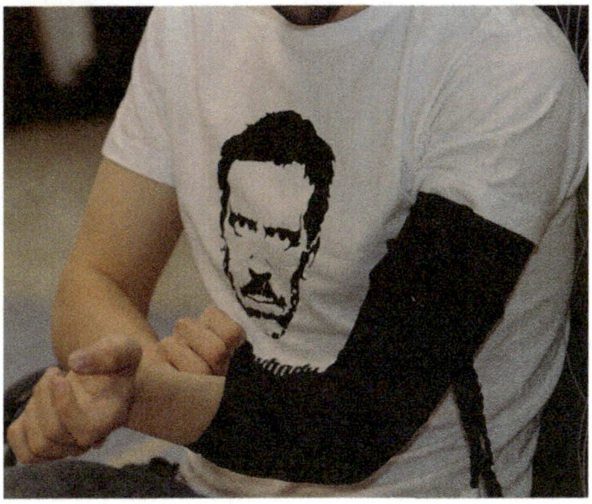

Fig. 6.5 Control subject wearing the conceptual TREMOR soft robot.

6.3.1 Development of Algorithms to Identify Intention to Move

The algorithm developed for the detection of voluntary motor activity from EEG signals is based on the real- time detection of the Event Related Desynchronization phenomenon, [62]. The algorithm is aimed at single-trial detection of voluntary movements. It first filters spatially the EEG signal by means of a surface Laplacian filter. The Laplacian filter is comprises C3, Cz, C4 electrodes and surrounding positions. The dereferenced data is then bandpass-filtered in two specific frequencies which are chosen based on the average desynchronization features obtained for each subject.

The power in these two frequency bands of interest is obtained in intervals of 25 ms in signal windows of 3s length. The estimated power value and the relation between two consecutive power values are used as input features for two Bayesian classifiers. The parameters of the probability distributions for the different features in the two classifiers are defined by the last 30 movements accomplished by the subject classified. Figure 6.6 illustrates the performance of the classifier in detecting the voluntary movement with the data from a patient.

6.3.2 Development of Algorithms to Identify Tremor Onset

First, a model of the surface EMG during tremor is developed. This model constitutes an attempt to combine neuromuscular models with biomechanical models and models of surface EMG generation, and serves as a tool for development of tremor modelling algorithms based on EMG activity. The complete model comprises two antagonistic muscles acting on a joint. Based on several types of synaptic input the motor neuron discharge pattern is estimated. The tremor is imposed by adding band-passed filtered white noise to the synaptic at any frequency and amplitude, allowing to vary the tremor. Muscle force and surface EMG are simulated based on this pattern, and the skeletal dynamics are estimated based on the force. The model is able to track any input angular trajectory for the limb.

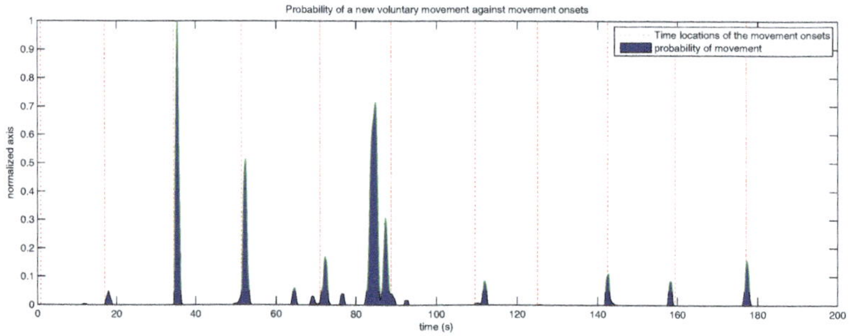

Fig. 6.6 Example of detection of tremor onset based on Event Related Desynchronization. The vertical lines represents the instants when movements occurred while the blue areas illustrates the probability of movement estimated by the Bayesian classifier.

According to the literature experimental data obtained during the recording sessions with patients, and simulated EMG from the above presented model, the research performed conclude that a feature of tremor EMG is a relatively clear spectral peak at the frequency of oscillation. On this basis, the algorithm to detect the onset of tremor is based on estimation of the power spectrum of the surface EMG. As pathological tremor exhibits frequencies in the range of 3-12 Hz, only this part of the power spectrum is used for the analysis. Once the power spectrum in this range is estimated, certain characteristics of the spectral peak are calculated; assuming that this would be the tremor frequency in case there is tremor in that particular muscle. Tremor detection is then based on fitting a Gaussian distribution around the peak to estimate its width, because tremor EMG typically presents a narrow peak when compare to no tremor EMG, Figure 6.7. This width is used as the detection parameter, by comparing it to a threshold value.

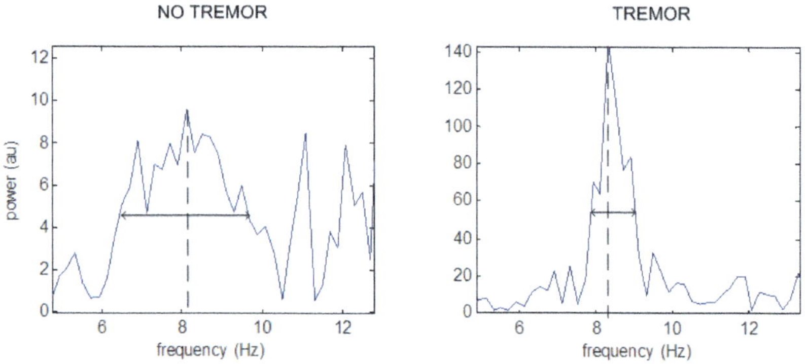

Fig. 6.7 The principle of the tremor detection algorithm using simulated surface EMG data. The width of the spectral peak is narrower in the case of tremor (right) compared to conditions with no tremor (left). The dotted line indicates the frequency with the highest power, and the arrow indicates the width of the spectral peak around this frequency.

This algorithm proves to be efficient, i.e. detect tremor onset without false positives in its absence, using length of data down to 1 s, at which point the poor resolution in the samples in the range of interest in each epoch would introduce significant bias into the detection.

6.3.3 Development of Algorithms for Tracking and Extraction of Tremor Characteristics

This section presents algorithms aimed at extracting instantaneous tremor amplitude and frequency from kinematic (IMU) information at joint level. The first step consists in characterizing joint rotations with IMUs. Differential measurement of a sensor placed distally with respect to the joint and another one placed proximally was implemented. Both sensors have one of their axes aligned with the users joint. The proposed algorithm for extraction of tremor parameters first separates tremor patterns from raw angular data, and afterwards estimates its instantaneous amplitude parameters. Real-time separation of voluntary and concomitant tremorous motion relies on their different frequency contents, whereas tremor modeling is based on an adaptive LMS algorithm and a Kalman filter, figure 6.8.

1. *Estimation of Voluntary Movement*: Estimation of voluntary movement is based on the fact that tremor alters voluntary motion in an additive manner, and that concomitant volitional movement during the activities of daily living (ADL) occurs in a frequency band lower than tremors. In fact, tremor is generally assumed to happen in the 3- 12 Hz band whereas ADL are performed at a frequency below 2 Hz. The implemented approach consists in modeling volitional motion as a first order process which is tracked with a Critically Dampened Filter, an optimal type of g-h tracker. Based on the additive nature of tremor, removing the voluntary component from the recorded joint rotation immediately yields the tremorous component of motion.
2. *Estimation of Instantaneous Tremor Parameters*: Estimation of instantaneous tremor parameters is implemented by means of two algorithms. First a Weighted Frequency Fourier Linear Combiner (WFLC) tracks instantaneous tremor frequency. This algorithm implements an adaptive Fourier model of the signal, which is adapted to the input signal based on the Least Mean Square (LMS) recursion, a gradient-like approach. Next a Kalman Filter that incorporates a harmonic model of tremor, estimates in- stantaneous amplitude taking into account WFLC frequency. The Kalman filter outperforms existing tremor modeling algorithms based on its intrinsic optimal nature.

Evaluation with data from the experimental session yielded an average tremor amplitude estimation error of 0.001 ± 0.002 rad/s (typical amplitude of tremor patients ranges between 1 and 2 rad/s), with frequency estimation in agreement with spectrograms, 6.8, [43].

Validation of tremor suppression strategies is being carried out in an iterative fashion. First, we have evaluated tolerance of tremor patients to FES in terms of

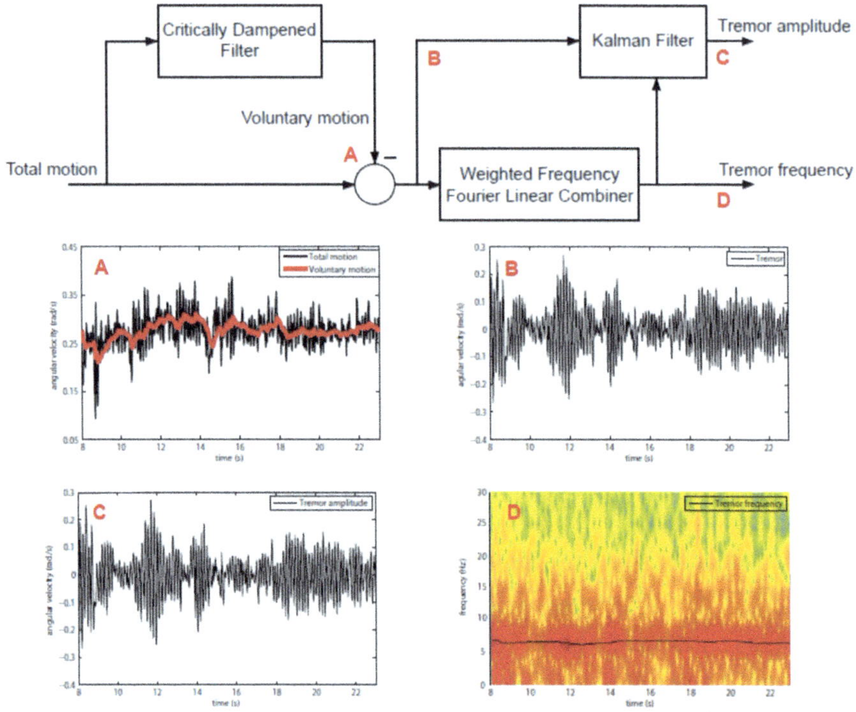

Fig. 6.8 Block diagram summarizing the two stage algorithm for estimation of instantaneous tremor parameters from IMU data. First, the algorithmgenerates an estimation of voluntary movement (A), that subtracted to the total motion provides an estimation of tremor (B). Next, tremor frequency is estimated with a Weighted Frequency Fourier Linear Combiner (WFLC), (D). Finally, a Kalman filter tracks instantaneous tremor amplitude based on the estimated tremor and the WFLC frequency (C).

discomfort and pain. Afterwards, we have studied the role that muscle FES induced fatigue plays in tremorogenic muscles. Next we have tested the impedance control strategy in open loop, i.e. with constant stiffness and damping increase. The impedance modulation strategy relies on modifyng the apparent joint stiffness and viscodity so that tremor is naturally filtered out, leaving concomitant voluntary movement unaffected. Considering that a human joint may be simply modelled as a second order system, [110], increased rigidity or damping decreases the cut off frequency of the low pass filter response of the joint, hence allowing for tremor attenuation. This is similar to the cocontraction strategiy employed by healthy subjects to stabilize the upper limb in a variety of situations, [54].

Preliminary results indicate that as expected results vary considerably among patient groups. Figure 6.9 shows attenuation of wrist tremor in an essential tremor patient while performing a postural task. Experimental results show migration of tremor to proximal joints when tremor is cancelled out through FES, supporting the need of independent joint controllers.

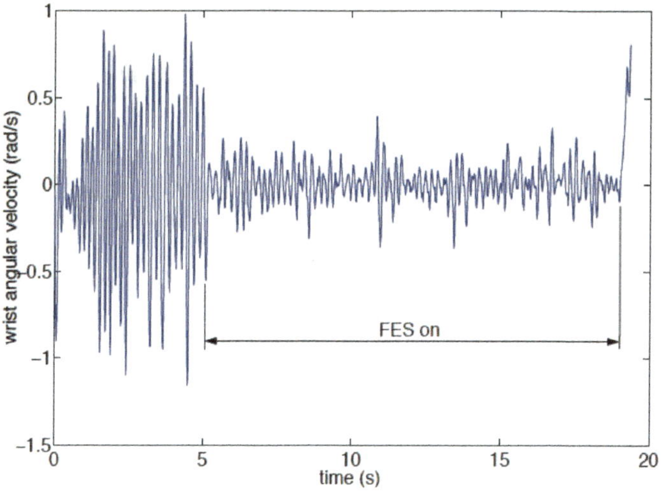

Fig. 6.9 Compensation of tremor in the case of an essential tremor patient keeping his arms outstrechted. During FES a considerable attenuation is observed, although tremor reappears when stimulation ceases.

Preliminary results with patients suffering from different types of tremor, though the results are yet preliminary, show the ability of the TREMOR neurorobot to model the generation, transmission, and execution of both volitional and concomitant tremorous movements. Moreover, these tests demonstrate the ability of the system to attain considerable attenuation of tremors. TREMOR concept will represent a step forward in different aspects of tremor suppression by means of FES:

1. It adopts for the first time a multi-joint FES approach (at least, wrist flexion-extension and adduction-abduction, forearm pronation-supination and elbow flexion-extension, according to the sensitivity analysis from DRIFTS).
2. The BCI-based detection, identification, characterization and tracking system is completely novel and will provide information on tremorous and voluntary motion and will allow us to be selective in the application of FES forces on only tremorous motion.
3. The combination of two mechanical suppression strategies (out-of-phase stimulation and modification of limb impedance) for a better management of most of the tremor types (rest, postural and kinetic).
4. For the first time, TREMOR concept aims at designing a garment-based embodiment totally wearable and compatible with normal human clothes. As a wearable device, it must exhibit a number of aesthetics, cosmetic as well as functional characteristics. To be accepted by potential users, the embodiment must be easy

to don and doff, so that the electrode and sensor placement be not an issue for the user.

5. The concept of TREMOR project will represent a step forward in BCI systems as it is intended to merge the information retrieved from both BCI-based sensors and limb motion sensors (IMUs) and in order to: detect the onset of tremor, distinguish voluntary and tremorous movement, and extract the time-varying characteristics of tremor movements, i.e. amplitude and frequency. The novelty of our concept is:

   - TREMOR will implement a self-training process through correlation of IMU-EMG, EMG-EEG information to avoid time consuming BCI training processes. This will also result in an adaptive system taking account of variability in EEG.
   - TREMOR will increase robustness of classical BCI systems through the use of redundant information at different stages of the neuromotor process: EEG-CNS, EMG-PNS and IMU-biomechanics. This will also have a positive impact on noise and artefact rejection.
   - Multimodality allows implementing self-evaluation of tremor management, not just on movement effects (tremor reduction) but on reorganization of neurophysiologic processes at both PNS and CNS levels.
   - Undesired effects on bioelectrical signals (e.g. cross talk of FES interference) is minimized.
   - TREMOR concept reduces computational burden as each modality is prone to provide different kinds of knowledge in a computationally inexpensive manner, i.e. EMG for tremor onset, EEG for intentionality of limb motion, IMUs for tremor amplitude and frequency. A truly Real Time system will be delivered.

6. TREMOR concept proposes a new methodology for FES, based on arrays of electrodes which overcome the limitations of actual electrodes for functional stimulation. In addition it will allow a more selective stimulation of muscles. The present project is focused in expanding these techniques together with the utilization of an innovative addressable electrode array system as a new approach to diminish fatigue. Moreover, these FES arrays improve comfort and reduce pain due to current distribution, i.e. the overall stimulation electric field will be set up in a summation process of painless and comfortable localized and distributed stimulations. In this regard, TREMOR will develop a multi-channel system that both stimulate and record EMG. This would be an important advance for FES in general and would go in the direction of minimizing the electrodes to locate on the subject.

This section presents the upcoming research in the development of a neuro-prosthetic solution for tremor suppression. These soft robots represents the next generation of robitcs in the rehabilitation field. In the future, the line separating the human and the robot will be fuzzier. In order to achieve this goal, robotics needs not only new technology, but also more science.

References

1. Adelstein, B.D.: Peripheral mechanical loading and the mechanism of abnormal intention tremor. PhD Thesis, Dept. of Mechanical Engineering, Massachusetts Institute of Technology (1981)
2. Aisen, M.: Glutethimide treatment of disabling action tremor in patients with multiple sclerosis and traumatic brain injury. Arch. Neurol. 49, 513–515 (1991)
3. Akay, M.: Biomedical signal processing. Academic, Sandiego (1994)
4. Akay, M.: Detection and estimation methods for biomedical signals. Academic, Sandiego (1999)
5. Alcantara, E., Forner, A., Ferrus, E., Garcia, A.C., Ramiro, J.: Influence of age, gender and obesity on the mechanical properties of the heel pad under walking impact conditions. Journal of Applied Biomechanics 18, 245–256 (2002)
6. American Medical Association, Guides to the evaluation of permanent impaired (1993)
7. Anouti, A., Koller, W.C.: Tremor disorders: diagnosis and management. The Western Journal of Medicine 162(6), 510–513 (1995)
8. Athalye, A.M.: Noth Filter Control of a Chaotic System. PhD thesis, Department of Mechanical and Materials Engineering, Washington State University, USA (1993)
9. EU Project CompanionAble, `http://www.companionable.net/` (last accessed, July 2010)
10. Bar-Shalom, Y., Li, X.: Estimation and Tracking: Principles, Techniques, and Software. Artech House Publishers, Boston (1998)
11. Battyke, C.K., Nightingale, A., Whilles Jr., J.: The use of myoelectric currents in the operation of prostheses. Journal of Bone and Joint Surgery 37B (1956)
12. Baydal, J.M., Barbera, R., Vivas, M.M., Sanchez-Lacuesta, J.J., Belda-Lois, J.M., Peydro, F., Prat, J., Gomez, A.: Analysis of the viscoelastic behaviour of the soft tissue response to external load and sensitivity map of the lower limb. In: International Journal of Rehabilitation Research: Proceedings of the 8th Congress of European Federation for Research in Rehabilitation, Ljubljana, Slovenia (2004)
13. Belda-Lois, J.M., Vivas, M.J., Castillo, A., Peydro, F., Garrido, J.D., Sanchez-Lacuesta, J., Barber, R., Poveda, R., Prat, J.: Functional Assessment of Tremor in the Upper-limb. In: Proceedings of the 8th Congress of European Federation for Research in Rehabilitation (2004)
14. Benedict, T.R., Bordner, G.W.: Synthesis of an optimal track-while-scan smoothing equations. IRE Trans. Automat. Control 7(4), 27–32 (1962)

15. Benito-Leon, J., Bermejo-Pareja, F., Morales, J.M., Vega, S., Molina, J.A.: Prevalence of essential tremor in three elderly populations of central Spain. Mov. Disord. 128, 389–394 (2003)
16. Bijak, M., Mayr, W., Rakos, M., Hofer, C., Ller, H., Rafolt, D., Reichel, M., Sauermann, S., Schmutterer, C., Unger, E., Russold, M., Kern, H.: The Vienna functional electrical stimulation system for restoration of walking functions in spastic paraplegia. Artif. Organs 26(3), 224–227 (2002)
17. Binder, D.K., Rau, G., Starr, P.A.: Hemorrhagic complications of microelectrode-guided deep brain stimulation. Stereotact. Funct. Neurosurg. 80, 28–31 (2003)
18. Blackman, S., Popoli, R.: Design and Analysis of Modern Tracking Systems. Artech House Publishers, Boston (1999)
19. Brookner, E.: Tracking and Kalman Filtering Made Easy. John Wiley & Sons, Inc., Chichester (1998)
20. Burkhard, P.R., Vingerhoets, F.J., Berney, A., Bogousslavsky, J., Villemure, J.G., Ghika, J.: Suicide after successful deep brain stimulation for movement disorders. Neurology 63, 2170–2172 (2004)
21. Caparros-Lefebvre, D., Blond, S., Vermesch, P.: Chronic thalamic stimulation improves tremor and l-dopa induced dyskinesias in Parkinson's disease. J. Neurol. Neurosurg. Psychiatry 56, 268–273 (1993)
22. Carroza, M.C., Laschi, C., Micera, S., Dario, P., Roccella, S., Carpaneto, J., Beccai, L., Pisetta, A., Odetti, L., Vechi, F., Mazzoleni, S.: Research on Rehabilitations Engineering at ARTS Lab, Scuola Superiore SantAnna, Pisa, Italy. In: Proc. of the 2007 IEEE 10th Inth. Conf. on Rehab. Robotics, NoordWijk, The Nederlands, June 12-15, pp. 590–600 (2007)
23. Chapin, J.K., Moxon, K.A.: Neural prostheses for restoration of sensory and motor function. CRC Press, Boca Raton (2000)
24. Cooper, G., Rodnitzky, R.: The many forms of tremor. Precise classification guides selection of therapy. Postgrad. Med. 108(1), 57–70 (2000)
25. Culmer, P., Jackson, A., Levesley, M.C., Savage, J., Richardson, R., Cozens, J.A.: An admittance control scheme for a robotic upper-limb stroke rehabilitation system. In: IEEE EMBS Annual International Conference, Shanghai, China, pp. 4028–4033 (2005)
26. Dallaway, J.L., Jackson, R.D., Timmers, P.H.A.: Rehabilitation Robotics in Europe. IEEE Transactions on Rehabilitation Engineering 3(1), 35–45 (1995)
27. Dario, P., Carrozza, M., Guglielmelli, E., Laschi, C., Menciassi, A., Micera, S., Vecchi, F.: Robotics as a future and emerging technology: biomimetics, cybernetics, and neuro-robotics in European projects. IEEE Robotics and Automation Magazine 12(2), 29–45 (2005)
28. Davis, B.J., OConnel, J.: Shoulder, elbow, and wirst components of physiologic tremor amplitude as measured using a laser pen light. European Neurology 43, 152–154 (2000)
29. Deuschl, G., Bain, P., Brin, M.: Consensus statement of the movement disorder society on tremor. ad hoc scientific committee. Mov. Disord. 13(3), 223 (1998)
30. Deuschl, G.: New treatment option for tremors. N. Engl. J. Med. 342(7), 505–507 (2000)
31. Edwards, R., Beuter, A.: A Using time frequency characteristics to discriminate physiologic and Parkinsonian tremors. Journal of Clinical Neurophysiology 16, 484–494 (1999)
32. Edwards, R., Beuter, A.: Using time domain characteristics to discriminate physiologic and Parkinsonian tremors. Journal of Clinical Neurophysiology 17(1), 87–100 (1999)
33. Elble, R.J., Koller, W.C.: Tremor. The Johns Hopkins University Press, Baltimore (1990)

34. Elble, R.J.: The pathophysiology of tremor. In: Watts, R.L., Koller, W.C. (eds.) Movement Disorders: Neurologic Principles and Practice, Koller WC, pp. 405–417. McGraw-Hill, Inc., New York (1997)
35. Elble, R.J.: Essential tremor frequency decreases with time. Neurology 55(10), 1547–1551 (2000)
36. Elble, R.J.: Characteristics of physiologic tremor in young and elderly adults. Clin. Neurophysiol. 114, 624–635 (2003)
37. Elble, R.J.: Tremor: Clinical Features, Pathophysiology, and Treatment. Neurol. Clin. 27, 679–695 (2009)
38. Eppinger, S.D., Seering, W.P.: Understanding bandwidth limitations in robot force control. In: Conference Proceedings 3rd IEEE International Conference on Robotics and Automation, Raleigh, USA, pp. 904–909 (1987)
39. Fahn, S., Tolosa, E., Marin, C.: Clinical rating scale for tremor. In: Tolosa, E., Jankovic, J. (eds.) Parkinsons disease and movement disorders, Urban & Schwarzenberg, Baltimore (1998)
40. Ferretti, G., Magnani, G., Rocco, P., Cecconello, F., Rossetti, G.: Impedance control for industrial robots. In: IEEE International Conference on Robotics & Automation, San Francisco, USA, pp. 4028–4033 (2000)
41. Friston, K., Frackowiak, R., Mauguire, F., Benabid, A.L.: Thalamic stimulation and suppression of Parkinson tremor. Evidence of a cerebellar deactivation using positron emission tomography. Brain 116, 267–279 (1993)
42. Fu, K.S., Gonzalez, R.C., Lee, C.S.G.: Robotics: Control, Sensing, Vision, and Intelligence. McGraw-Hill Book Company, New York (1970)
43. Gallego, J.A., Rocon, E., Roa, J.O., Moreno, J.C., Pons, J.L.: Real- time estimation of pathological tremor parameters from gyroscope data. Sensors 3, 2129–2149 (2010)
44. Gao, J.B., Wen-wen, T.: Pathological tremors as diffusional processes. Biological Cybernetics 86, 263–270 (2002)
45. Goonetilleke, R.: Designin to minimize discomfort. Ergonomics in Design, 12–19 (1998)
46. Gonzalez, J.G., Heredia, E.A., Rahman, T., Barner, K.E., Arce, G.R.: Filtering involuntary motion of people with tremor disability using optimal equalization. In: Proc. of the 1995 IEEE Int. Conf. on Systems, Man and Cybernetics (1995)
47. Gonzalez, J.C., Garca, A.C., Vivas, M.J., Ferris, E., Alcantara, A., Forner, A.: A new portable method for the measurement of pressure-discomfort threshold (ptd) on the foot plant. In: Proceedings 4th Symposium on Footwear Biomechanics, Canmore, Canada (1999)
48. Gresty, M., Buckwell, D.: Spectral analysis of tremor: understanding the results. J. Neurol. Neurosurg. Psychiatry 53, 976–998 (2000)
49. Hallet, M.: Classification and treatment of tremor. JAMA 266, 1115–1117 (1991)
50. Harwing, W.S., Rahman, T., Foulds, R.A.: A review of design issues in rehabilitation robotics with reference to North America research. IEEE Transactions on Rehabilitation Engineering 3(1), 3–13 (1995)
51. Harwin, W.S., Leiber, L.O., Austwick, G.P.G., Dislis, C.: Clinical potential and design of programmable mechanical impendances for orthotic applications. Robotica 16, 523–530 (1998)
52. Hendriks, J.: A second-generation joystick for people disable by tremor. In: Proc. 14th Annual RESNA Conf., pp. 248–251. Ed. RESNA Press, NY, Elmsford (2002)
53. Hogan, N.: Mechanical impedance control in assitive devices and manipulators. In: Proceedings of the JACC, p. TA10B, San Francisco, CA (1980)

54. Hogan, N.: Impedance control: An approach to manipulation: Part I - theory. Journal of Dynamics System, Measurement and Control 107, 17 (1985)
55. Hogan, N.: Impedance control: An approach to manipulation: Part II - implementation. Journal of Dynamics System, Measurement and Control 107, 8–16 (1985)
56. Hogan, N.: Impedance control: An approach to manipulation: Part III - applications. Journal of Dynamics System, Measurement and Control 107, 17–24 (1985)
57. Hogan, N.: Estable execution of contact tasks using impedance control. In: Proceedings of IEEE International Conference on Robotics and Automation, vol. 2, pp. 1047–1054 (1987)
58. Hollerbach, J.M.: Workshop on the design and control of dextrous hands. MIT-AI Memo No. 661 (1982)
59. Hollerbach, K., Kazerooni, H.: Modeling human arm movements constrained by robotic systems. Advances in Robotics ASME 42, 19–24 (1992)
60. Holmes, G.: The symptoms of acute cerebellar injuries due to gunshot injuries. Brain 40, 461–535 (1917)
61. Huang, N.E., Shen, Z., Long, S.R., Wu, M.C., Shih, H.H., Zheng, Q., Yen, N.-C., Tung, C.C., Liu, H.H.: The empirical mode decomposition and the Hilbert spectrum for non-linear and non-stationary time series analysis. In: Proc. Roy. Soc. Lond., vol. 454, pp. 903–995 (1998)
62. Ibáñez, J., Serrano, J.I., del Castillo, M., Barrios, L.: An asynchronous BMI system for online single-trial detection of movement intention. In: Proceedings of the 32nd Annual International Conference of the IEEE Engineering in Medicine and Biology Society (2010)
63. Inoue, T.: Practical repetitive control system design. In: Proc. 29th IEEE Conf. Decision Control, vol. 3, pp. 1673–1678 (1990)
64. Jain, S.S., Kirshblum, S.C.: Movement disorders, including tremors. In: Joel, A., DeLisa, J.B. (eds.) Rehabilitation Medicine: Principles and practice, vol. 2. Lippincott Company, Philadelphis (1993)
65. Johnson, G.R., Carus, D.A., Parrini, G., Scattareggia, S.R., Valeggi, R.: The design of a five degree-of-freedom powered orthosis for the upper limb. In: Proceedings Instn. Mech. Engrs., vol. 25 (2002)
66. Kalman, R.: A new approach to linear filtering and prediction problems. ournal of Basic Engineering - Transactions of the ASME Journal 82, 35–45 (1960)
67. Kapandji, I.A.: The physiology of the joints: Upper limb. Churchill Livingstone (1983)
68. Astrom, K.J.: Introduction to control. Department of Automatic control, Lund University (2002)
69. Kazerooni, H.: Human–Robot Interaction via the Trnasfer of Power and Information Signals. IEEE Transactions on Systems, Man and Cybernetics 20(2), 450–463 (1990)
70. Koller, W.C., Busenbark, K.L.: Essential tremor. In: Watts, R.L., Koller, W.C. (eds.) Movement Disorders: Neurologic Principles and Practice, pp. 365–375. McGraw-Hill, Inc., New York (1997)
71. Kotovsky, J., Rosen, M.J.: A wearable tremor-suppression orthosis. J. Of Rehabilitation Research and Development 35(4), 373–387 (1998)
72. Krebs, H.I., Dipietro, L., Levy-Tzedek, S., Fasoli, S.E., Rykman-Berland, A., Zipse, J., Fawcett, J.A., Stein, J., Poizner, H., Lo, A.C., Volpe, B.T., Hogan, N.: A paradigm shift for Rehabilitation Robotics. IEEE Engineering in Medicine and Biology Magazine, 61–70 (July/August 2008)
73. Krouskop, T., Krebs, M., Herskowicz, I., Graber, S.: Effectiveness of mattress overlays in reducing interface pressure during recumbency. Journal of Rehabilitation Research and Development 22, 7–10 (1985)

74. Kwee, H.M.: Rehabilitation Robotics - Softening the Hardware. IEEE Engineering in Medicine and Biology, 330–335 (1995)
75. Leva, P.: Adjustments to zatsioorsky-seluyanovs segment inertia parameters. Journal of Biomechanics 29(9), 1223–1230 (1996)
76. Lippold, O.J.C., Redfearn, J.W.T., Vuco, J.: The rhythmical activity of groups of motor units in the voluntary contraction of muscle. J. Physiol. 137, 473 (1957)
77. Louis, E.D.: Behavioral symptoms associated with essential tremor. Adv. Neurol. 96, 284–290 (2005)
78. Louis, E.D., Honig, L.S., Vonsattel, J.P., Maraganore, D.M., Borden, S., Moskowitz, C.B.: Essential tremor associated with focal nonnigral Lewy bodies: a clinicopathologic study. Arch. Neurol. 62, 1004–1007 (2005)
79. Lu, Z., Goldenberg, A.A.: Implementation of robust impedance and force control. Journal of Intelligence and Robotic Systems 2, 145–163 (1992)
80. Mann, K., Werner, F.W., Palmer, A.K.: Frequency spectrum analysis of wrist motion for activities of daily living. Journal of Orthopedic Research 7(2), 304–306 (1989)
81. Manto, M., Topping, M., Soede, M., Sanchez-Lacuesta, J., Harwin, W., Pons, J.L., Williams, J., Skararup, S., Normie, L.: Dynamically responsive intervention for tremor suppression. IEEE Eng. Med. Biol. 22(3), 120–132 (2003)
82. Manyam, B.V.: Uncommon forms of tremor. In: Watts, R.L., Koller, W.C. (eds.) Movement Disorders: Neurologic Principles and Practice, pp. 387–403. McGraw-Hill, Inc., New York (1997)
83. Manzoni, D.: The cerebellum implement the appropriate coupling of sensory inputs and motor responses: evidence from vestibular physiology. Cerebellum 4, 178–188 (2005)
84. Maples, J.A., Becker, J.J.: Experiments in force control of robotic manipulators. In: Conference Proceedings 2nd IEEE International Conference on Robotics and Automation, San Francisco, USA, pp. 695–702 (1986)
85. Markenscoff, X., Yannas, I.V.: On the stress-strain relation for skin. Journal of Biomechanics 12(2), 127–129 (1979)
86. Lawrence, J., Marple, S.: Computing the discrete-time analytic signal via fft. IEEE Transactions on signal processing 47(9), 2600–2603 (1999)
87. Mason, M.: Compliance and force control for computer controlled manipulators. IEEE Transactions on Systems, Man, and Cybernetics 11(6), 418–432 (1981)
88. Maurel, W.: 3D Modeling of the human upper limb including the biomechanics of joints, muscles and soft tissues. PhD Thesis (1998)
89. Michaelis, J.: Introducing the neater eater. Action Res. 6(1), 2–3 (1988)
90. Morrell, J.B., Salisbury, J.K.: Parallell-coupled micro-macro actuators. The International Journal of Robotics Research 17(7), 773–791 (1998)
91. Moreno, J.C., Rocon, E., Ruiz, A.F., Brunetti, F., Pons, J.L.: Design and implementation of an inertial measurement unit for control of artificial limbs: application on leg orthoses. Journal of Sensors & Actuators B 118, 333–337 (2006)
92. Pledgie, S., Barner, K.E., Agrawal, S.K., Rahman, T.: Tremor suppression through impedance control. Tremor suppression through impedance control 8(1), 53–59 (2000)
93. Pratt, G.A., Williamson, M.M., Dillworth, P., Pratt, J., Ulland, K., Wright, A.: Stiffness isnt everything. In: Proceedings of the 4th International Symposium on Experimental Robotics, Stanford, CA, USA (1995)
94. Pons, J.L.: Emerging Actuator Technologies. A Micromechatronic Aproach. John Wiley & Sons, Chichester (2005)
95. Pons, J.L.: Wearable Robots: Biomechatronic Exoskeletons. Churchill Livingstone (2008)

96. Popovic-Bijelic, A., Bijelic, G., Jorgovanovic, N., Bojanic, D., Popovic, M.B., Popovic, D.B.: Multi-field surface electrode for selective electrical stimulation. Artif. Organs 29(6), 448–452 (2005)
97. Popovic, M.R., Keller, T.: Modular transcutaneous functional electrical stimulation system. Med. Eng. Phys. 27(1), 81–92 (2005)
98. Popovic, D.B., Sinkjaer, T.: Neuromodulation of lower limb monoparesis: functional electrical therapy of walking. Acta neurochir. 97(1), 387–393 (2007)
99. R Development Core Team R: A Language and Environment for Statistical Computing. R Foundation for Statistical Computing (2006)
100. Rabischong, P.: Robotics for the handicapped. In: Proceedings IFAC Control Aspects of Prosthetics and Orthotics, pp. 163–167 (1982)
101. Raibert, M.H., Craig, J.J.: Hybrid position/force control of manipulators. ASME Journal of Dynamic Systems, Measurements and Control 102, 275–282 (1981)
102. Rahman, T., Sample, W., Seliktar, R., Alexander, M., Scavina, M.: A body-powered functional upper limb orthosis. Journal of Rehabilitation Research and Development 37(6), 675–680 (2000)
103. Randall, J.E.: A stochastic time series model for hand tremor. J. appl. Phys. 34, 390–395 (1973)
104. Ratanaswasd, P., Dodd, W., Kawamura, K., Noelle, D.: Modular behavior control for a cognitive robot. In: Proceedings of the 12th International Conference on Advanced Robotics, pp. 713–718 (2005)
105. Riley, P.O., Rosen, M.J.: Evaluating manual control devices for those with tremor disability. Journal of Rehabilitation Research and Development 24(2), 99–110 (1982)
106. Riviere, C.: Adaptive suppression of tremor for improved human-machine control. PhD thesis. Johns Hopkins University, Baltimore (1995)
107. Riviere, C.N., Rader, R.S., Thakor, N.V.: Adaptive Cancelling of Physiological Tremor for Improved Precision in Microsurgery. IEEE Transactions on Biomedical Engineering 45(7), 839–846 (1998)
108. Rocon, E., Belda-Lois, J.M., Sanchez-Lacuesta, J.J., Pons, J.L.: Pathological Tremor Management: modelling, compensatory technology and evaluation. Journal of Technology & Disability 16, 3–18 (2004)
109. Rocon, E., Ruiz, A.F., Pons, J.L.: On the use of ultrasonic motors in orthotic rehabilitation of pathologic tremor. In: Proc. of ACTUATOR 2004 Conference, XIX, MP30, pp. 387–390 (2004)
110. Rocon, E., Ruiz, A.F., Pons, J.L.: Biomechanical modelling of the upper limb for robotics-based orthotic tremor suppression. Applied Bionics Biomechanics 2(2), 81–85 (2005)
111. Rocon, E., Ruiz, A.F., Pons, J.L.: On the use of rate gyroscopes for tremor sensing in the human upper limb. In: Proceedings of the International Conference Eurosensors XIX, MP30 (2005)
112. Rocon, E., Belda-Lois, J.M., Sanchez-Lacuesta, J.J., Ruiz, A.F., Pons, J.L.: Estimation of biomechanical characteristics of tremorous movements based on gyroscopes. In: Asistive Technology - from Virtuality to Reality, Lille, France, AAAT 2005 (2005)
113. Rocon, E., Andrade, A., Pons, J.L., Kyberd, P., Nasuto, S.: Empirical mode decomposition: a novel technique for the study of tremor time series. Medical & Biological & Engineering & Computing 44, 569–582 (2006)
114. Rocon, E., Ruiz, A.F., Pons, J.L., Belda-Lois, J.M., Snchez-Lacuesta, J.J.: On the use of an active wearable exoskeleton for tremor suppression via biomechanical loading. In: Proceedings of the 2006 IEEE International Conference on Robotics and Automation (2006)

115. Rocon, E., Belda-Lois, J.M., Ruiz, A.F., Manto, M., Pons, J.L.: Design and Validation of a Rehabilitation Robotic Exoskeleton for Tremor Assessment and Suppression. IEEE Transactions on Neural Systems and Rehabilitation Engineering 15(3), 367–378 (2007)
116. Rosen, M., Arnold, A., Baiges, I., Aisen, M., Eglowstein, S.: Design of a controlled-energy-dissipation orthosis (cedo) for functional suppression of intention tremors. J. of Rehab. Research and Develop. 32(1), 1–16 (1995)
117. Roy, J.: Force controlled robots: Design, analysis, control and applications. PhD Thesis. John Hopkins University, Baltimore, MD, USA (2001)
118. Roy, J., Whitcomb, L.L.: Adaptive force control of position/velocity controlled robots: theory and experiments. IEEE Transactions on Robotics and Automation 18(2), 121–137 (2002)
119. Salisbury, J.K.: Active stiffness control of a manipulator in cartesian coordinates. In: Proceedings of the 19th IEEE Conference on Decision and Control, Albuquerque, NM, USA, pp. 95–100 (1980)
120. Salisbury, J.K., Craig, J.K.: Articulated hands: Force control and kinematic issues. International Journal of Robotics Research 1(1), 4–17 (1982)
121. Schmitt, O.: Some interesting and useful biomimetic transforms. Third International Biophysics Congress 297 (1969)
122. Scholtz, J.C.: Human-robot interactions: creating synergistic cyber forces. In: Proceedings of the NRL Workshop on Multi-Robot Systems, pp. 177–184 (2002)
123. De Schutter, J., Van Brussel, H.: Compliant robot motion II. a control approach based on external control loops. Int. J. Robot. Res. 7(4), 18–33 (1988)
124. Sharma, R., Pavlovic, V.I., Huang, T.S.: Toward multimodal human-computer interface. Proceedings of the IEEE 5(86), 853–869 (1998)
125. Stein, R.B., Oguztreli, M.N.: Tremor and other oscillations in Neuromuscular systems. Biological Cybernetics 22, 147–157 (1976)
126. Stiles, R.N.: Mechanical and neural feedback factors in postural hand tremor of normal subjects. J. Neurophysiol. 44(1), 40–59 (1980)
127. Surdilovic, D., Vukobratovic, M.: Control of robotic systems in contact tasks. In: Nwokah, O.D.I., Hurmuzlu, Y. (eds.) Mechanical Systems Design Handbook: Modeling, Measurement and Control. CRC Press, Boca Raton (2001)
128. Gantert, G., Honerkamp, J., Timmer, J.: Analysing the dynamics of tremor time series. Biological Cybernetics 66, 479–484 (1992)
129. Timmer, J., Lauk, M., Pfleger, W., Deuschl, G.: Cross-spectral analysis of physiological tremor and muscle activity: I Theory and application to unsynchronized electromyogram. Biological Cybernetics 78, 349–357 (1998)
130. Timmer, J., Huler, S., Lauk, M., Lcking, C.H.: Pathological tremors: Deterministic Chaos or non-linear stochastic oscillators? CHAOS 10, 278–288 (2000)
131. Townsend, W.T., Salisbury, J.K.: The effect of coulomb friction and stiction on force control. In: Conference Proceedings 3rd IEEE International Conference on Robotics and Automation, Raleigh, USA, pp. 883–889 (1987)
132. Tsagarakis, N.G., Caldwell, D.G.: Development and control of a soft-actuated exoskeleton for use in physiotherapy and training. Autonomous Robots 15, 21–33 (2003)
133. Van der Loos, H.F.M.: VA/Stanford Rehabilitation Robotics research and development program: lessons learned in the application of robotics technology to the field of rehabilitation. IEEE Transactions on Rehabilitation Engineering 3(1), 46–55 (1995)
134. Vodovnik, L., Bajd, T., Kralj, A., Graanin, F., Strojnik, P.: Functional electrical stimulation for control of locomotor systems. Crit. Rev. Bioeng. 6(2), 63–131 (1981)

135. Ushe, M., Mink, J.W., Revilla, F.J., Wernle, A., Schneider Gibson, P., McGee-Minnich, L., Hong, M., Rich, K.M., Lyons, K.E., Pahwa, R., Perlmutter, J.S.: Effect of stimulation frequency on tremor suppression in essential tremor. Mov. Disord. 19, 1163–1168 (2004)
136. Velthuis, W.J.: Learning Feed-Forward Control: Theory, design and applications. PhD thesis, University of Twente, The Netherlands (2000)
137. Villani, L., de Wit, C.C., Brogliato, B.: An exponentially stable adaptative control for force and position tracking of robor manipulators. IEEE Trans. Automat. Contr. 44, 778–802 (1999)
138. Vincent, J.F., Bogatyreva, O.A., Bogatyrev, N.R., Bowyer, A., Pahl, A.K.: Biomimetics: its practice and theory. Journal of the Royal Society, Interface / the Royal Society 3(9), 471–482 (2006)
139. Whitney, D.E.: Force feedback control of manipulator fine motions. ASME Journal of Dynamic Systems, Measurements and Control 99, 91–97 (1977)
140. Wu, M., Abbott, J.J., Okamura, A.M.: Effects of velocity on human force control. In: First Joint Eurohaptics Conference and Symposium on Haptic Interfaces for Virtual Environment and Teleoperator Systems (World Haptics), pp. 73–79 (2005)

Batch number: 10837190

Printed by Printforce, the Netherlands